„A Lithium Life" by Marcus Maure

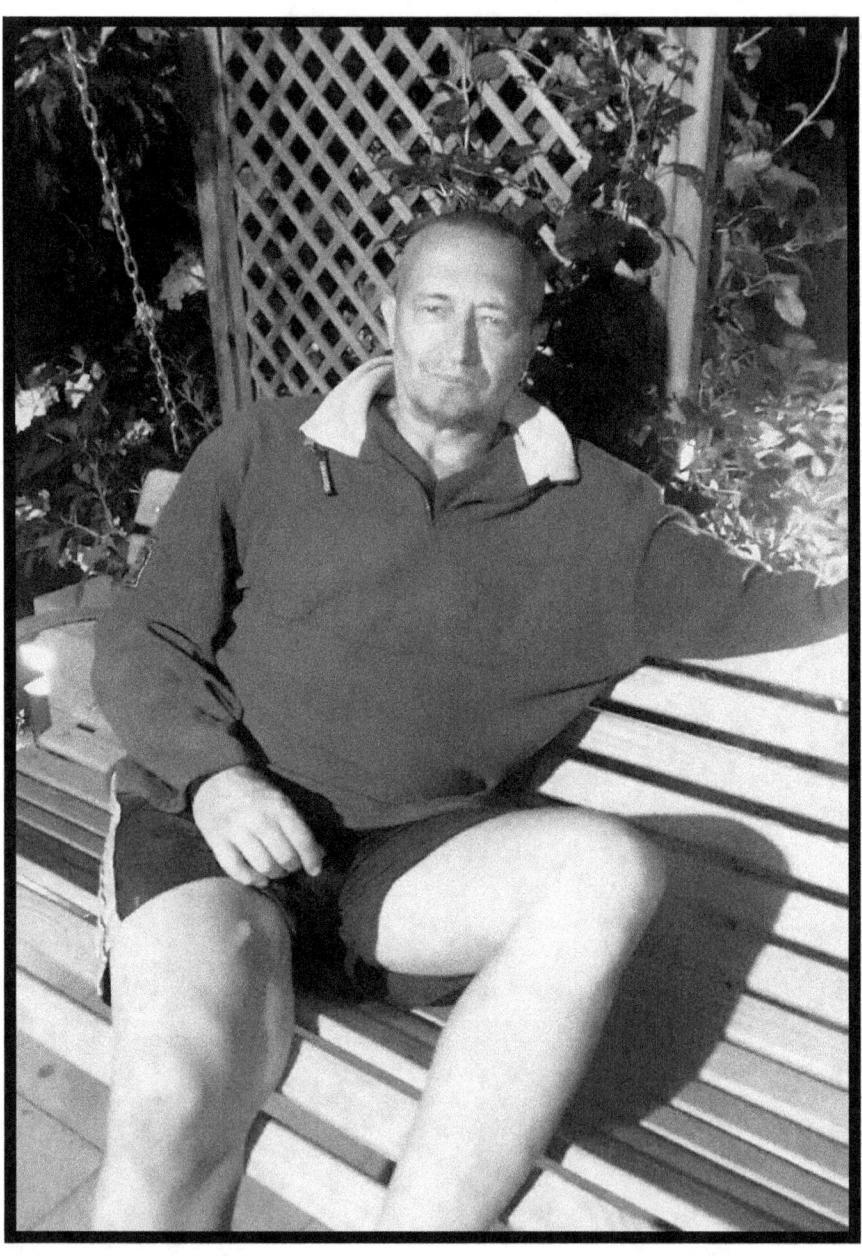

All rights reserved. No part of this book may be reproduced or distributed in any form without prior written permission from the author, with the exception of non-commercial uses permitted by copyright law.

No part of this book may be reproduced or transmitted by any means, except as permitted by UK copyright law or the author. For licensing requests, please contact the author at keithm7272@gmail.com

All rights reserved. No portion of this book may be reproduced, copied, distributed or adapted in any way, with the exception of certain activities permitted by applicable copyright laws, such as brief quotations in the context of a review or academic work.

For permission to publish, distribute or otherwise reproduce this work, please contact the author at keithm7272@gmail.com

Contents

Introduction 5
Chapter 1 - The gene pool 10
Chapter 2 - Leaving East Africa 19
Chapter 3 - My mum 23
Chapter 4 - My formative years 28
Chapter 5 - Growing up 51
Chapter 6 - End of the line 62
Chapter 7 - Here comes the rain... again 74
Chapter 8 - From pillar to post 82
Chapter 9 - The power of love 91
Chapter 10 - Self admission to a psychiatric ward 101
Chapter 11 - Going home 111
Chapter 12 - Moving out and moving on 119
Chapter 13 - Living the dream 125
Chapter 14 - An early sign of trouble 139
Chapter 15 - The next few years 149
Chapter 16 – Loving life, generally 157
Chapter 17 - What just happened? 177
Chapter 18 - Monday morning blues 184
Chapter 19 – The Phoenix rises 193
Chapter 20 - Polska here I come 203
Postscript 210

Introduction

My name is Marcus Maure; I was born in January 1963 in Frimley in Surrey, England. I have lived with bipolar disorder for almost as long as I can remember. Bipolar disorder used to be more commonly known as manic depression, but as this title associated the illness with the highly stigmatized label of the "maniac", its name was changed to bipolar disorder in the 1980's.

The British Psychological Society (BPS) website defines bipolar disorder as a **mood disorder**. The term itself is a contraction of two words: "bi" meaning two, and "polar" standing for opposite or extreme sides. So, does pretty much is what it says on the tin.

The disorder is thought to be caused by an imbalance of the chemicals that are responsible for controlling the brain's functions, these neurotransmitter chemicals include noradrenaline, serotonin and dopamine. Having bipolar disorder is strongly linked to genetic influences as an inherited condition, and it is the most common psychiatric condition to be passed down through the family.

The BPS site explains that bipolar disorder causes changes to one's mood, usually consisting of shifts between extreme high (mania) and low (depressive) moods. They explain the two states as exhibiting the following characteristics or symptoms**:**

Signs of mania:

    Increased energy

    Excitement

    Impulsive/reckless behaviour

    Agitation

    Aggressiveness

Signs of depression:

    Decreased levels of energy

    Feelings of worthlessness

    Feelings of hopelessness

    Difficulty in concentrating on an activity

    Loss of interest in activities

    Low self-esteem and suicidal thoughts

I would like to add two further personal comments about this illness: firstly, that **it is** an illness and the mood swings are not necessarily predictable or as a consequence of the sufferers behaviours or lifestyle (although these factors can play a role); and secondly, depending on the severity, being in either of the two extreme states can be debilitating and crippling; drastically affecting the person's ability to function effectively and cope with even the simplest daily routines and responsibilities. In the effective treatment/management of the condition a combination medication approach is frequently required, using drugs which aim to help regulate the patient's mood swings, and different medication to try and address the extreme aspects of the manic or depressive states e.g. psychosis, hypomania. In my case, after some trial and error, a combination of lithium salts and fluoxetine (branded as Prozac) appears to work best for me.

On a more positive note, living with bipolar disorder is of course doable, particularly with treatment. Approximately 1 in 100 people will be diagnosed as having bipolar at some point during their lives (with many more affected but never receiving a diagnosis) and go about their daily business, in the main, quietly and possibly at times, not so quietly, functioning adequately in their different societal roles e.g. parent, partner, employee, boss, friend, neighbour. Many famous celebrities have/had bipolar disorder such as: Stephen Fry; Russell Brand; Carrie Fisher; Buzz Aldrin; Katherine Zeta-Jones; as well as successful business people, entrepreneurs and leaders including: Theodore Roosevelt; Winston Churchill; and more contemporarily Elon Musk and Ted Turner. It is quite likely that some of the more manic aspects of their bipolar condition, such as their never-ending flow of creative ideas, their perseverance and determination and of course their high energy levels and increased appetite for risk have played a crucial part in contributing to their success.

I just wanted from the get go, to give those of you unfamiliar with this illness, a quick crash course on the condition and to hopefully demystify it a little bit. As I mentioned, only a few decades ago I, and other sufferers, would have been labelled with the scary title of "a manic depressive", which is likely to have instinctively made you wary of me. And do I want to reassure you on behalf of myself and others with this condition, that whilst we may be mad we're not crazy.

What follows is my account and reflections on the people and events that have shaped my life and in particular the impact of living with my bipolar condition. You will hear about my repeated cycling from manic phases to depressive states, sometimes with long periods of relative stability in between. I have had at least four significant breakdowns, during which I was reduced to levels of functioning in which I was just about able to get through each day (often only with help from others), and I have been hospitalized (voluntarily) twice to help me through the worst of the lows. Having written this book what I am more convinced about than ever, is that many of the life changing actions, and decisions I have made, which resulted in great successes or catastrophic failures, were taken during times when I was either in or entering into a manic or depressive phase. My current stability and happiness, which still feels precarious at times, has not come easily and has not been plain sailing. This will come as no surprise to any readers who themselves have or have lived with someone who is bipolar, or for that matter any other debilitating mental health condition. Although I haven't beaten the illness, I first started taking medication for my condition when I was in my late teens and I will be on it for the rest of my life (my occasional attempts at taking myself off my meds have shown this to be not a good idea for me), I have survived, and at times even thrived as a result of my illness. I have learned to live with my condition; it does not define who I am, although at times it has brought me to my knees and taken me close to my limits.

I now live in Wroclaw in Poland, with my Polish wife, our two wonderful teenage sons and our four much loved (but noisy) dogs. I also have a beautiful and successful daughter Joanne (Jo), from my previous short marriage to Caroline in the UK. I earn my living by teaching English to Polish businesses and by actively managing my modest investment portfolio. In recent years it has been far more common for Polish citizens to move to the UK, than my migration the other way and although I have lived here now for 25 years (a quarter of a century!), I will admit it was not a move I ever anticipated making; never really part of my life plan. It just sort of happened as a solution at the time to a set of circumstances and events that had left me on a downward life trajectory, one from which I needed to escape, to take time out, to reset and to hopefully rebuild myself and my life.

My name is Marcus Maure, I have bipolar disorder and this is my story:

Chapter 1 - The gene pool

The Family

Tessa (my mother)

Sonny/Dad (my grandfather)

Agnes/Nana/Agi (my grandmother)

Yolah, Vernon, Stennie and Richard (my uncles and aunts)

Sonny

My grandad, Donovan Stanford Maure, known to his friends as Sonny, was born in Nairobi in 1910. I don't know too much about his family, although I think he had two siblings - a brother and a sister. Sonny had a modest upbringing, and ironically although he himself was something of an English Loyalist, his father fought for the Germans in the First World War. Sonny's father died while Sonny was still a boy, and whether this was a factor or not, Sonny never attended formal school. Sadly, Sonny's mother became blind in later life and he spent what spare time he had looking after her. The rest of his time he devoted to his passion and fascination, automobiles, and from his early teens he started helping out in a local garage as a mechanic's assistant. Sonny soon became a skilled mechanic, learning by doing, and developing a particular expertise in repairing the model T- Ford automobiles that were ubiquitous at that time in many African countries. Sonny joined the British

Army and fought for King and Country in some of the Colonial Wars and uprisings that were common in Africa at that time. Based mainly in Africa as a mechanic in a Tank Regiment, he saw active service during World War 2, which thankfully he managed to survive without injury. After the War he returned to Tanganyika (now part of modern Tanzania) and started working for a large rubber plantation. He rose swiftly through the ranks to become chief engineer, a position he held for many years. Sonny was highly intelligent, self-educated and he taught himself to speak four languages fluently; English, French, Italian and Swahili (it is ironic that in his later years when he withdrew into himself, he didn't speak much in any language). In Africa he was a hardworking man, well respected in the community he lived, and he spent a lot of his leisure time at the Colossal Club where he met my grandmother, Agnes, whom he affectionately referred to as Agi. They married, had five children, and lived a comfortable, privileged, colonial lifestyle; subsidised by his employer, who provided the family with a company house and servants. Comfortable enough for them to be able to educate all of their children privately.

Agi

Agnes or Agi (Agi means fire in Sanskrit), my dear grandmother, was born in the Seychelles in 1915 and was raised by her mother and her father, the latter who worked for the British Post Office. Agnes was educated at a French convent school and spoke mainly French when she was growing up. She was also fluent in English, except when in one of her frequent states of "excitability" when her strong accent and mispronunciation of many words would render her virtually unintelligible in any language. My grandmother moved with her family to Africa when her father was posted there with his job, and there she met, fell in love with and married my grandfather. Agi took responsibility for raising their five children and running the household whilst Sonny was out at work, a task that must have been made a lot easier for her with the help of seven servants that she had somehow acquired. Although she had no formal employment whilst in Africa, Agi set about the work of managing her household in an authoritarian and business-like manner. She used her sharp tongue to great effect in directing and overseeing her servants' activities, an approach which resulted in her being alternately loved and feared, but always obeyed. Her scolding manner was a constant feature throughout her life and woe betide the poor servant who failed to carry out their cleaning duties to the required standard. They would be singled out, publicly humiliated with a public exposition of their failings and told in no uncertain terms that their position and status in life was a sign of God punishing them for not being of White Anglo-Saxon Protestant heritage. She was certainly a product of her time and situation.

Despite her apparent insensitivities and her autocratic management style, Agi could also show great concern and care towards her servants at times. If any of them had a sick child she would immediately go to their home with food and medical supplies, and on the occasions when approached by unemployed locals unable to put food on their table, Agi would take them in and give them work. This last point probably explains why she had seven servants to help her manage a household that must have been well ordered most of the time since her five children were away at private school. No doubt this benevolent (sometimes malevolent) matriarch induced confusion and mixed emotions amongst her staff's feelings and loyalties, and I can only presume it was this ambiguity that saved her at times from being lynched by an uprising from within her own household.

Whilst it is more common for an individual to have both maternal and paternal grandparents, or at least to have some knowledge and understanding of their existence, unfortunately and regrettably, I never met or knew anything about my father and consequently I have nothing to add here about my paternal grandparents. On reflection, in the total absence of a father, a mother who was an erratic and unreliable influence in my life (much more on her later), and maternal grandparents who struggled practically and emotionally with the realities of their less privileged post-colonial life in the UK, perhaps a second set of grandparents with a different set of perspectives and histories might have been a positive influence for me. Although, given the track record of the blood relatives I did know about, perhaps not!

At the time, living in Africa with a husband who worked long hours away, children at private school, and a house that miraculously seemed to keep itself clean (although the seven servants may have begged to differ with the last point), my grandmother had plenty of opportunity to look for other distractions to occupy her time. This high energy, volatile time bomb of a woman needed to be kept busy and occupied for her own state of mind as well as for the well-being of all those around her. Agnes found that she had two innate skills which she turned to in helping her fill her days: the first was that she appeared to have the gift of clairvoyance, and the second was that she really enjoyed cooking, particularly the making of curries.

My grandmother developed her clairvoyance skills with the help of her African friends, particularly the local community elders. She used this talent in Africa, and later in the UK, to give psychic readings and tell people their futures and fortunes. She did this both freely and for money, the latter more so in the UK when the household income was much more precarious and where her customers were more able to cross her palm with silver. One of the stories passed down by my uncle Vernon was that my grandmother sometimes used a Ouija board to help her summon up the spirits in her clairvoyance sessions. On one such occasion when the glass was moving around the board seemingly propelled by some psychic force, she had asked out loud if anyone from the spirit world was listening! At which point the table lifted itself of the ground and flew violently against the wall, smashing to pieces... I guess that counted as a "yes". After this event my grandmother made a vow never to summon the spirits using the Ouija board ever again, judging that this was bad juju indeed.

Although only about knee high to a grasshopper Agi's combative nature meant that she loved nothing better than a fight, usually verbal but on occasion verging on the physical; and the local food markets in the African villages frequently provided the perfect battleground. Vernon told of another (presumably traumatic but comical in the retelling) embarrassing childhood memory when he was out shopping with his mother on one occasion. Having wandered off on his own he heard his mother's shouts and rushed over in the direction of her voice. He found her engaged in a stand-up quarrel with another customer in the fish market. Amid a small crowd that had gathered, the two antagonists each had one end of a huge fish, one the head and the other the tail, and were pulling the fish backwards and forwards, neither willing to let go as they fought over ownership. My uncle did not say who won out on the day, although I know who my money would have been on.

My grandmother's hysterical shouting and screaming at all and sundry was a constant feature of family life, and she and Sonny would often resort to shouting at each other in French like in some bizarre farce of "not in front of the children", not appreciating that all 4 children were well versed in French as a result of their private school education. My grandmother's multilingualism was also used to comic effect whenever she was revealing bad information or gossip as she would say out loud "attention petites orielles" (attention little ears) which the children found very funny.

Life in the immediate environment outside the family home in Africa could also be challenging and dangerous. The family had a house dog, in part for protection and also as a family pet; he was a Rhodesian Ridgeback called Red. My mother loved the dog very much and was traumatised when tragically one night, Red was attacked and killed by a leopard that had wandered into their garden. It seemed that Africa provided a potentially hostile environment for my mother and her siblings both within and without the confines of the Maure household.

By now you should be building a picture of the formidable character that was my grandmother, and in spite of her diminutive stature (or maybe because of it) the confrontational approach she adopted in most aspects of her life. She didn't limit her hysterical behaviour to the confines of her household either, and whether at home giving the servants a tongue lashing, or in the village markets haggling over the price and quality of potential purchases, she had a boundless supply of nervous energy that needed (and thankfully was) venting regularly. I can almost hear the village stall holders' knees knocking and scurrying for cover when the word went out that Agi was in town on her weekly shopping trip. Dear Nana, she was an unlikely source of humour, but the recounting of these stories brings a smile to my face.

The Maure children

As the Maure children came of age, for various reasons, most notably the pursuit of their own careers and relationships, they began returning to the UK. Richard, who was the most talented and gifted of the children, had to give up a place at Chelsea Art College because his wife Bryony had become pregnant, and so he needed to earn some regular income to support his family. He turned to a career in tailoring, and became a very good suit maker for Burtons, settling down to family life in Camberley in Surrey. My Aunty Yolah moved to the west country and set up home in Launceston in Cornwall with her husband Peter. They had two children, Jeffrey and Jennifer, and many of my early childhood memories are of visiting them in what felt like an idyllic existence. No doubt this view would have been coloured in part by the fact that those visits were when I was on vacation, during summer holidays when school was out.

I consider my Uncle Vernon to be the closest person to a father I ever knew. Vernon and his brother Stennie, had both been required to do National Service; Vernon joined the elite paratrooper corps and Stennie joined an Army infantry regiment. To avoid a return to the family home in Africa and also as a way of continuing to earn a reasonable wage, Vernon extended his service with the Paras after National Service and trained as a para-medic. He loved this role and thrived under the military lifestyle in Aldershot, progressing to the rank of Staff Sergeant.

My mother Tessa was always my grandparent's favourite. Together with her sister, Yolah, she was provided with all the benefits and luxuries her parents could afford, whilst living the high life in Africa. Tessa was her parent's pride and joy, which must have felt unfair and difficult for Yolah, who was judged second in all things by comparison to her prettier, more confident, and more precocious younger sister. My mother was sent to a convent at an early age for her schooling, and then on to a finishing school in Belgium. I am unsure how much this elitist education, away from her parents influence, helped her in reality, or even if it contributed in some way to the poor mental health she suffered from throughout her adult life. She went on to make two suicide attempts (or at least two that we knew of), the second one being successful; successful for her at least as it did provide her with relief from the torment she felt in living.

My Aunty Yolah on the other hand, didn't go to finishing school, she wasn't sent anywhere. Presumably my grandparents didn't feel that her potential warranted the lavish investment they had made in her sister. Instead Yolah met and married a lovely man who I got to know very well, Peter Tregarthen. Peter had a great affinity with animals, including pets and livestock, and although not formally trained in any way, he carried out the duties of a vet in the African village community. At the first opportunity after they married, Yolah and Peter escaped Africa (and my grandmother's influence) and went to the UK where Peter had secured a position as the manager of a petrol station, and the two set about establishing a household of their own. Very sadly though, by this time Peter, who had always been a heavy drinker, had succumbed to alcoholism and he went downhill fast. He became incapable of managing the business and was drinking what little profits it made. He and Yolah divorced shortly after returning to England. I remember Peter very fondly, as he regularly came to stay for extended periods with my grandparents and me in Frimley Green. By this time, he was more a ghost than a person, a shadow of his former self, rarely speaking and more often than not, curled up sleeping in an alcoholic stupor underneath items of household debris on the sofa in our front room. His dejected presence alongside that of my depressed grandfather must have been a struggle for my grandmother.

Chapter 2 - Leaving East Africa

In 1962 after my grandmother had contracted yellow fever for a second time, the doctors advised my grandparents that they should move to a cooler climate for the sake of my grandmother's health. So, the remaining family took the drastic step of uprooting themselves and moving to the UK, where my grandfather bought a small house for £3,000 in Frimley Green, a little village on the Surrey/Hampshire border. It must have been very difficult for the family to adjust to this radical relocation and the consequent change to their lifestyle, I imagine it a bit like Gerald Durrell's family's move to Corfu in „My Family and Other Animals", but in reverse. They swapped a privileged colonial lifestyle and the variety an African landscape for a small semi-detached in the grey and nondescript English suburbs, although on the upside at least the family pets were far less likely to be eaten by leopards in Frimley Green. My grandfather's mechanical and engineering experience served him well; aged around 50 he quickly got a job as fitter with the National Gas and Turbine Establishment ("NGTE", part of the Royal Aircraft Establishment), making gas turbines and jet engines for aircraft. Although this was a skilled position, it was not a patch on the responsibility and status that he had given up on the plantation in Tanganyika. He spent the remainder of his official working career at the NGTE, retiring at the age of 65. His company pension would have allowed him to retire earlier aged 60, but the prospect of spending all his time at home with Agi (their relationship had not got any less tempestuous) resulted in him choosing to work the additional five years. Throughout my grandparent's married life there does seem to be a pattern in which Sonny spent as much time as he could away from the family home and the fiery Agi, either working all the available hours on the plantation in Africa, working beyond his company retirement age at the NGTE, or subsequently spending the majority of his post retirement days at the Conservative Club. This distance from each other was probably the secret of my grandparent's long marriage, although my grandmother did her best to make up for lost time with her constant barrage of shouting at Sonny on the occasions when he did make an appearance at home.

My grandparent's small semi-detached house was far from grand; blink and you would miss it as you drove past on the main road towards Aldershot. Bizarrely, for a house of its modest stature, some former owner had felt strongly enough about it to give it a name „Pyecombe", and it had something of a disturbing past. The previous owner, a man called Charlie, had hanged himself in the small orchard in the back garden and according to my grandmother, Charlie's spirit was present all throughout the house (this might in part explain the very low £3,000 price tag). Being sensitive to the psychic world, my grandmother said that Charlie came to her frequently in her dreams. There were also mysterious knocks at the backdoor, which revealed no one there when opened, and we all regularly heard unexplained noises in the night. Fortunately, I didn't learn about the house's past until I was a bit older, otherwise I would have been terrified.

Another talent that my grandmother possessed was the ability to play multiple, as many as 10, bingo cards simultaneously, a skill she honed over time at the Colossal Club in Africa. The thrill of the risk and possible gain from this early low stake form of gambling stayed with her throughout her life and she remained throughout a regular (but modest) gambler. Perhaps she viewed this habit as a chance to contribute to the household finances, which since moving to the UK had proven a lot more challenging to manage, and they constantly robbed Peter (metaphorically of course... not my Uncle Peter) to pay Paul when it came to settle the most pressing debts. As a young boy I remember that everything we bought seemed to be on tick or credit. We seemed to owe money to each of the village shops; the newsagents, the food store, and the off-licence would all get paid at the end of each month. Even our larger purchases and clothes were bought on credit through a home purchasing system from a company called Blundells and a man would come around each week (the tallyman or the knockerman) to collect our payments. My grandmother became one of Blundells' star customers, and they reciprocated by keeping a seemingly limitless line of credit available to her. My grandfather, theoretically the head of the household, appeared totally oblivious or disinterested in these goings on. Although I couldn't have put a name to it then, I realise now that since leaving Africa, he had suffered with a depression that resulted in him rarely participating in any of the activities and decision making in the house. Mentally he was still living his life out in Africa in the bush and surviving on memories and nostalgia. His new reality was watching the news and constantly reading books that he would borrow from the library, just around the corner. History was his favourite subject, primarily war, and there was a suspicion that he had a secret admiration for Germany's Nazi leader, Adolf Hitler. Sonny appeared able to put to one side Hitler's faults (of which I think we can agree he had one or two) as he respected the leadership, vision and genius he showed when it came to making war (at least perhaps in the early years of World War 2). Understandably these views resulted in my grandfather often being teased about his alleged sympathies during family get togethers, primarily from his sons who were both by then serving in the British Army.

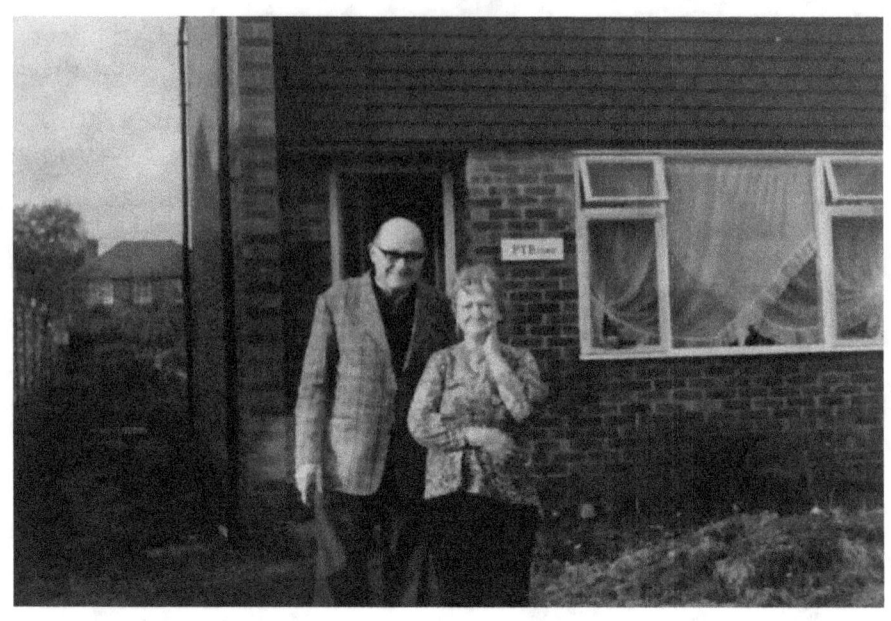

My grandparents outside their house in Frimley Green.

Chapter 3 - My mum

By now Tessa, my mother, had returned from her Belgian finishing school and was looking for a job in England. Not surprisingly she found it difficult to live under the same small roof as her constantly quarrelling parents and instead she spent a lot of time staying with my Uncle Vernon and Auntie Myra in Aldershot. Myra took my mother under her wing and generally looked out for her. One night at a party Tessa was introduced through one of Myra's friends to a man named David. She became close to David and they started seeing each other romantically. It was from this relationship that my mother became pregnant and I came into existence. David, a man who I know next to nothing about, have never met or even seen a photo of, is my father, and sadly, very much a bit player in my story. Okay, well that's enough about "Dad". Tessa, who was then only 19, decided she wanted to have and keep the baby (thanks for that, Mum), perhaps her Catholic upbringing and the church's views on abortion had something to do with her decision. Anyway, she gave birth to me on the 27th of January 1963 at Frimley hospital and went with her new-born child to live with her parents at Pyecombe in Frimley Green; which is when and where I enter the story.

London life

Having taken the decision not to terminate but to have the baby, the reality was that my mother's lifestyle and ambitions were not at all compatible with the task of raising a child. In Africa she had been subject to a strict upbringing by her parents, something which continued under the nuns in the Catholic finishing school in Belgium. As such this young woman's opportunities for fun had been few and far between and it is not surprising that upon her move to the UK she was drawn to the highlife and thrill of London, which was now virtually on her doorstep. Together with a friend of hers called Jean, Tessa moved into a flat in Kensington, only a short bus ride to Oxford Street where she had got a job in the perfumery department at Selfridges, the prestigious department store. My mother's outgoing nature and good looks were her greatest social assets in London and she soon found herself living in a world of clubs and parties, unlike anything she could have dreamed of in Africa. She was the epitome of a good-time girl at the centre of perhaps the most exciting city in the world at the dawn of the swinging sixties. Her looks brought her some modelling work and, in this environment, she met several would-be suiters. She dated rich, famous, and influential people including celebrities and TV stars. One significant relationship she had around this time was with a man called Jimmy S, who owned several successful restaurants in London. I can remember as a very small boy being taken to feed the ducks with my mother and „Uncle Jimmy" as I was encouraged to call him. As a child, I had more "uncles" than I could count due to the constant stream of new boyfriends entering and departing my mother's life). I imagine that in her efforts to be a responsible mother, each new beau was introduced to me early on; a litmus test if ever there was one. Anyway, for some reason this memory of feeding the ducks with my mother and Jimmy, or was it Bob or David? .... sticks firmly in my mind.

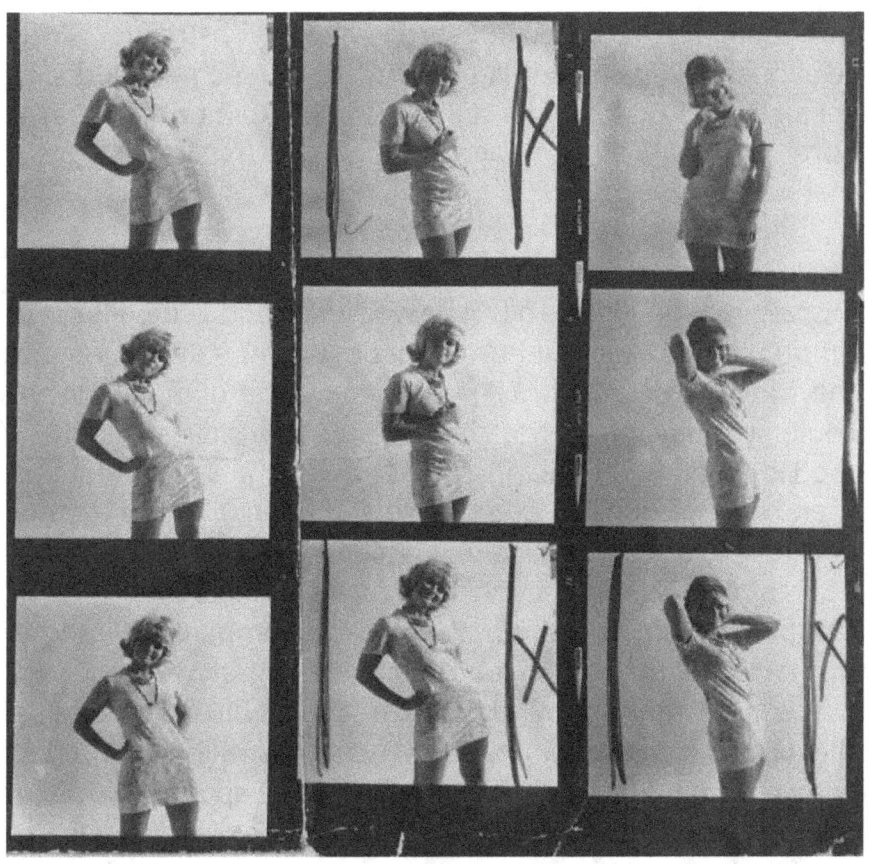

<u>Tessa's attempts at a modelling career.</u>

I was wrong before when I said I would say no more about my father, and I may have encouraged the wrong impression about his character based on his lack of involvement with me. After my mother became pregnant, I am told my father's family were very supportive and offered to look after me when I was born; actively encouraging their son's relationship with my mother. Apparently, David a tall, well-educated man with a promising career working in the ophthalmic industry was particularly keen on pursuing a long-term relationship with my mother and bringing me up as his son. But Tessa, still only 19 and already with a taste of the high life, had different plans. By this time, she had become tired of the constraints of her relationship with David and wanted to pursue her modelling career in the big City, which is when she split up with David. Sorry David... Dad, I hope that puts the record straight.... thanks for trying.

Occasionally my Uncle Vernon would visit his youngest sister Tessa, in London to see how she was doing and generally check up on her. On one visit having made a cup of tea, he went to the fridge looking for milk; on opening the door all that he could see were bottles of champagne, no visible signs of any food, or sadly any milk - just the bare essentials. My mother's friend Jean seemed to exert a strong influence on my mother, and I remember when visiting once when I was about seven years old noticing how posh mum now sounded; speaking as if she had a plum in her mouth. In Jean's company my mother appeared to try and imitate her speaking style, something which I personally found strange and a bit embarrassing. Maybe this is a case of my child's memory seeking to find fault with a mother who had chosen to live a life apart from me, or maybe despite my mother's outward confidence it reflects that she felt the need to adapt her personality in order to fit better with the society and socialites she was now mixing with.

At that time, at such a young age, I was of course unaware of my mother's instability, oblivious to her bouts of depression and the occasions when she had overdosed on pills. I was however conscious that wherever my mother went she brought with her drama and excitement (hysteria even). Somehow this vibrancy and craziness seemed an important part of her appeal to many of the men she dated; I think they must have sensed her vulnerability and wanted to look after her and protect her. What seems slightly creepy to me now is that I recall that most of the men she went out with were considerably older than she was, Jimmy Smalley for example was closer to my grandfather's age, maybe as much as 30 years older than my mother (I sometimes wonder just what it was they had taught her at that Belgian finishing school).

Chapter 4 - My formative years

Soon after I was born, the constant friction and tension between my grandparents and my mother, caused in part from all living together (plus baby me) in what must have been a febrile atmosphere under the same small roof at Pyecombe, had become too unbearable for my mother to keep coming back to be with me and instead she decided that it would be for the best if I was placed into temporary foster care. In her jumbled thinking she rationalised that in the future when she was stable and secure enough, her lifestyle less chaotic, and she was living together with her perfect partner, I would return to live with her (presumably in this aspirational future there would also be milk and food as well as Champagne in her fridge). I am told that at that time, Myra and Vernon offered to adopt me, but my mother rejected this idea as it ran counter to her dreams of a future in which mother and child would once again live together under the same roof. If anyone had asked me for my opinion back then, I would have jumped at the chance of becoming part of my aunt and uncle's family; I loved them both dearly and I was very close to their children, my cousins, Julie, and Chris.

And so, for a period of time I was fostered into a very nice family with a foster mother called Sylvia who had two children of her own. I have good memories of staying there and playing with the children within an environment that was calm, happy and stable, compared to the goings on in my grandparent's house. This turned out to be only a brief respite however because although nothing had changed within my own family, i.e. my mother was still emotionally unstable, showed no sign of getting her act together, and continued to have a number of short term relationships, the period of fostering ended abruptly and I went back to Frimley Green. It transpired that my grandparents had agreed to adopt me and become my legal guardians. I can only assume that the relevant authorities had determined that they were fit to take on this role based on the evidence of how well they had brought up their own children! How on earth did they think my grandparents would be able to bring me up on their own and without the help from 7 servants! From this point onwards to minimise confusion for myself and external parties I started calling my grandfather "Dad" and my grandmother "Nana", but in these pages I shall continue to refer to them as my grandfather and grandmother so as not to confuse.

Following my return to my grandparents I began again seeing my mother a lot more regularly. Her mood had lifted and she appeared to have re-found her boundless energy and she wanted to spend as much time with me as she could. In terms of her life priorities, I was to come second only to her career and lifestyle in London (hmmm?). At this stage in my mother's life, if we refer to the points made earlier about the classic characteristics of the bipolar condition, she was moving from a period of depression into a manic phase. She would come back from London to see me in Frimley Green two or three times a week, and in addition I would often visit and stay with her in London at the weekends where I met lots of her friends and boyfriends (honorary uncles) and generally have a great time. I guess I found her buoyant mood during this period infectious and intoxicating, and I worshipped and adored this vivacious young woman who I remember feeling lucky enough to have as my mother. I loved those weekends, and the fact that sometimes on a Saturday morning I would wake up in my bed to find that my mother had come back late on the Friday evening and was lying in bed asleep next to me; what better surprise could there possibly be for a young boy. I am not blind to my mother's faults and weaknesses, but I know that she loved me back and endeavoured to put me at the centre of her life.

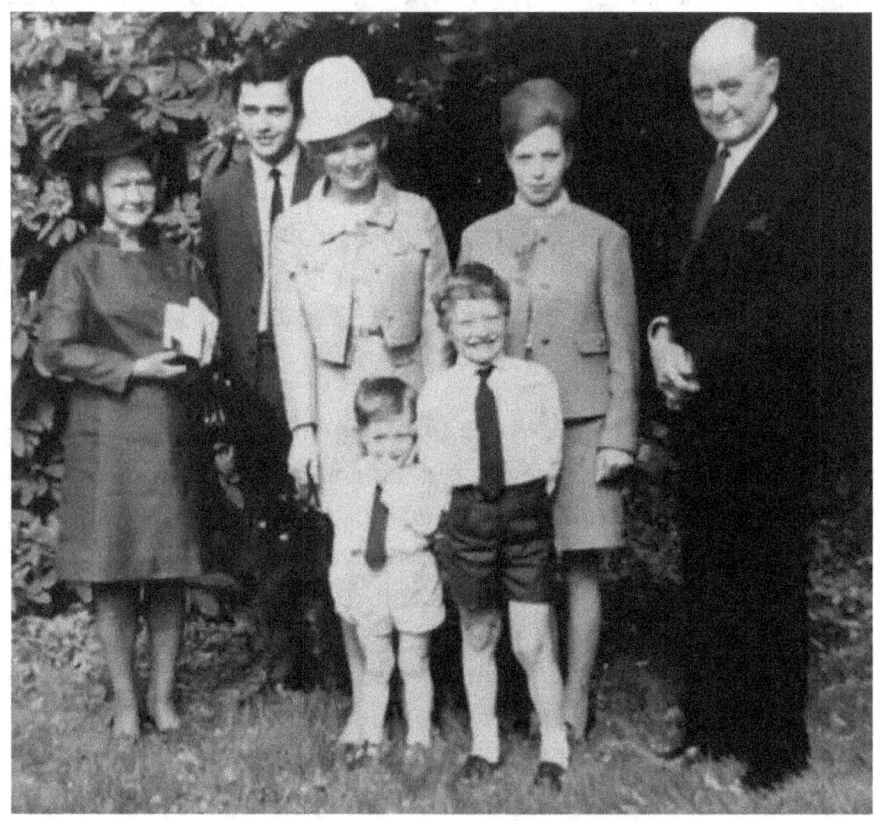

Quite a nice photo of me with my mum, grandparents, Uncle Richard and his wife Bridey with my cousin Clinton (the smaller boy) on my first Holy Communion (looks like I'm entering a manic phase)

In many ways I was lucky. My mother loved me, my grandmother doted on me, and at that time it seemed that everyone went out of their way to be nice to me. My grandmother fussed over me all the time although my grandfather remained rather distant. By then he had become something of a passenger in the house, not taking part in anything that was going on, preferring instead to inhabit the fond memories in his head of his life in Africa, and a time when he had status and respect. Now living in this alien country at a stage in his life when by all rights he had earned an entitlement to some peace and tranquillity he found himself in a very chaotic environment with his high maintenance wife, manic youngest daughter, and lo and behold an adopted grandchild to boot – living the dream! That is not to say that he didn't try on occasion; I remember happy times when he worked alongside me using his mechanical skills to help me fix my push bikes and motorcycles.

Meanwhile my mother and my grandmother seemed to be constantly vying for my affections, pulling me in different directions; just like the fish in the African market (and we know how that turned out), both were over-compensating for my lack of a normal family upbringing, with the predictable result being that I was definitely becoming spoiled. Their behaviour's wakened in me some innate child's awareness that I possessed an emotional power over them both which I could, and did, use to manipulate things to my benefit. I began to use this new-found power to my advantage (or so I misguidedly thought) by feigning frequent stomach aches when I didn't want to go to school, which was quite often in those days. One such bogus stomach ache lasted six weeks and resulted in my grandmother, who I had convinced of my condition, allowing me to stay at home all that time until there came an inevitable knock at the door by a woman from the social services enquiring as to why I wasn't at school: sadly my powers of manipulation and emotional blackmail had little effect on her.

Perhaps as a result of this incident, my school life was to take an unexpected turn for the better. Dimpner, a friend of my grandmother's from Church, suggested to her that perhaps as we were Catholic (me in name only) she should consider sending me to the local Catholic school, St Tarcisius in nearby Camberley. And so one day I went to visit the school with my mother and whilst she talked to the headmaster in his room, I sat on some steps in the hallway sobbing with crocodile tears because hey guess what?... Little Lord Fauntleroy doesn't want to go to this school either! I can only surmise that I had exceeded the limit of my emotional manipulation since at the start of the very next term I found myself at St Tar's in class Infant 4. I didn't realise it then but this introduction to the Catholic community and Church would later play a significant part in my adolescent life.

From my first day at St Tar's I became friendly with Tom Bartlett, another boy from my village, as we both travelled together on the school bus from Frimley Green. Tom was the son of our local GP, Dr Bartlett, and Tom's mother ran the local playschool out of their big house, which was right next to the village green. The Bartletts were widely considered an eccentric and highly intelligent lot, Tom being no exception to this rule. Not only was he bright, quick and intelligent, Tom soon developed an ability to turn a profit on the back of his talents. One great example of this was when in his late teens, Tom was making a killing (relatively) playing a general knowledge-based quiz machine in the local pubs. The particular machine was based on the TV snooker show," Pot Black". Tom's knowledge of trivia and the arcane, combined with his instant recall and his canny strategizing made the challenge an unequal contest, and in this battle, man (well, boy actually) consistently outsmarted machine, time and again. Unfortunately for Tom, word soon got around to the local publicans and before long he was banned from playing the machines in all the pubs in Frimley Green. Tom being Tom just shrugged his shoulders, took a puff on his pipe (yes, a pipe smoker in his late teens) and moved onto the next village's pubs and some other way to use his "smarts" towards making some easy money.

Anyway, back at my new school St Tar's, I sat next to Tom, as he was the only person I knew. I cannot explain why but this time school felt very different; I quickly began to enjoy myself and looked forward to going there each day. My previous inconsistent attendance had taken its toll though and I found myself playing catch up in most subjects including the basics of reading, writing and arithmetic. I remember with some embarrassment fairly soon after starting at St Tar's, we were set a multiple-choice test of about 40 questions. As usual I was sat next to Tom who, sensing my apprehension, sagely advised me „don't think too much, I find it best to go with my first instinct". I followed Tom's advice to the letter and proceeded to answer all the questions within the space of five minutes, finishing ahead of anyone else. What I had not appreciated was that Tom's advice and confidence in his own strategy worked for him since crucially, it was built upon his extensive general knowledge. To Tom it was just like the pub quiz game, although I don't think at that age even he had yet started playing on them. My approach however was based entirely on Tom's advice and completely randomised guesswork with zero underpinning knowledge. Needless to say, I got the lowest mark in the class and Tom of course, who finished only slightly after me, came top.

My greatest enjoyment in that first year was play-time. We had two 15-minute play times and an hour for lunch, although in the case of the latter a lot of time was taken up in queueing for and eating lunch. But there was still time to play football or conkers or to get involved in the occasional fight with boys from different classes. My school experiences were becoming like those of most kids of my age; at last I was leading a more normal life. St Tar's was not a particularly large school, it mainly serviced the large Irish Catholic population from the nearby Old Dean Estate, but there were enough kids of the same age to require some in year streaming based on ability. This produced one memorably poignant moment for me when returning to school at the end of the summer holiday after my first year. During the holidays I had become even firmer friends with Tom having spent hours playing together on the green. On the first day back, I followed Tom to the classroom and took up my customary position, seated at the desk beside him. When the teacher finally looked up, to my horror she addressed me out loud in front of the class and told me that I was in the wrong class and should instead be next door (in the next academic stream down). I felt greatly humiliated as I had to get up and leave the class, knowing that this was as good as announcing publicly to everyone that I was not as clever as they were.

Just in case you are feeling too sorry for me at this point I should point out that other aspects of my life, particularly my domestic arrangements, were going fantastically and I was having a ball. Together with my resurgent mother I had just been taken on an outing to an aerodrome with Jimmy Smalley, during which I had been treated to a ride in the rear passenger seat of a vintage two-seater aeroplane. Very exciting for a small boy but terrifying at the same time and something that I wouldn't necessarily choose to repeat again. I was spending a lot of time in London visiting the various great parks, including Hyde Park where on hot days I could swim and paddle in the Serpentine. I did notice, even then, that my mother seemed happier and less moody during the summer, somehow stronger and more robust and resilient to the challenges she faced in her daily life. This is something that I shared with her as I am at my best during the warm months between May and September.

Like most boys back in the early 1970s, I spent a lot of my free time out riding my bike or playing football on the village green. These good times began to provide me with a more solid and contented base for my general development and consequently combined with increased attentions to my studies; I made good academic progression particularly in maths and science. This maturation included noticing and becoming more aware of girls, and now in addition to us boys playing football, we would take time out to start playing and fooling around with the girls as a means of getting to know them and to be noticed by them more. Oh, those birds and those bees, they would have a lot to answer for!

The golden years

These were certainly proving to be my halcyon days; my social life had come on in leaps and bounds through my sporting endeavours - I joined my local football club Mytchett Athletic, and I progressed to play for the school first team in the left-wing position, that of my hero and world superstar Georgie Best. Playing for the school team had a real kudos attached to it even at that age and marked you apart from the other kids. This fact was evidenced by the boys who were in the school team who wore their school shirts with pride at every possible sporting opportunity, as if to publicise their elite status. What made this all the funnier is that the school football shirts in question (I remember a combination of sky blue and navy blue colours) were the tattiest, scruffiest, moth eaten garments you could ever imagine, in reality little more than rags. Most of the positional numbers, which were displayed on white cotton squares stitched to the back of the shirts, were literally hanging off. But that didn't matter; it was what the shirt represented and said about the wearer that mattered: "I am in the school team, I am to be admired". I find it difficult to imagine this happening today when young kids (or more likely their parents) every season happily fork out close to a hundred pounds for an authentic kit of their favourite team; probably purchasing both home and away strips. Would they instead don a garment that was barely recognisable as a shirt and looked as if it had just been used to clean the floor with? Well, we did, and I would do so again to relive that same God-like feeling.

Anyway, I digress, where was I? Oh yes, these were truly wonderful and glorious times in my childhood blah blah blah. My mother was going through a relatively stable period which meant I saw her a lot and she prioritised her attention towards me. She was by now living with a new man called Alan. Alan was a divorcee with a 16/17 year old son Mark, who was a talented artist, and who on my weekly visits introduced me to the cool music he was listening to. Alan was a banker and lived in Richmond and had been divorced from his wife for several years. It was clear to me that he doted on my mother and really cared about her. Sadly, for him, for me, and perhaps for my mother as well, he quickly became yesterday's news as far as my mother was concerned when another man with a flashier car, a material asset that consistently seemed to appeal to my mother's need for excitement and the extravagances of wealth, came along. Then there was Ernest, another restauranteur who drove an Aston Martin. I often found school parents evenings awkward as I had to bear the embarrassment of my very vocal, eccentric grandmother shouting out loud and once again I would find myself explaining why my dad was my grandad, and where was my real mum and dad! Lines of questioning that I found mortifying and excruciating to deal with and always tried desperately to avoid. But nothing could top my enjoyment than the time my mum turned up to one parents evening with Ernest in his Emerald Green Aston Martin DBS, and I climbed into the back seat in front of the envious eyes of hundreds of gawking schoolchildren. I could tell that my mother was also well aware of these looks and probably took a little too much reflected glory from the envy that she saw in them.

Life at home during this period was, if not normal, then at least reasonably constant and predictable; my mother visited regularly and we had great times going to Aldershot Lido during the hot summer months when she and the weather were at their best. School was good, and my social life was full with friends and fun. Added to this I was being well loved and looked after by my grandmother who ensured there was always a nourishing meal on the table for me and had by then started helping me with my French homework. By contrast my grandfather wasn't doing much apart from sitting on the sofa, rolling tobacco, watching the news, and reading his many war books. Slowly the state of the house was beginning to deteriorate and in the front room there was now a circle of yellow stained ceiling directly above where he sat and smoked in front of the fire. But I wasn't about to let a little bit of front room dinginess get me down as I certainly had no intention of inviting any friends home to witness my grandmother's incessant tirades hurled at my grandfather for being a „lazy bastard." Also, around this time my grandmother was receiving two or three strangers a day who visited the house to have their fortunes told. These clairvoyance sessions were bringing in quite a bit of money and of course they also provided her with the opportunity to talk to someone new. My grandfather and I, in some unspoken agreement of solidarity, were both grateful that at least for the duration of these visits she had a distraction from nagging at either of us.

Although we never seemed to have much money, we must have been managing okay, since in 1973 we started renting a colour TV from Vision Hire for £7.95 per month. This must have taken a significant slice of the household budget, but I had eventually worn my grandmother down with my constant whining. Up until only a few years previously we hadn't even had a fridge in the house and in all the time I lived there we never had central heating. Our approach to heating the house had instead been to install a gas fire in the front room, in the belief that the heat would permeate upwards, nicely warming the remainder of the small house. In reality what happened was that we got subtropical temperatures in the living room and arctic conditions upstairs. However, thanks to some strategic purchases of calor gas heaters and electric blankets from good old Blundells, we managed to get through the cold winters. As I write this I am reminded of how different, strange even, my home life was from those of my friends in their centrally heated homes with all their mod cons, and their conventional family structures, but there is no doubt about it – at that time I was having a ball.

Things were about to change again in my mother's love life; this time she moved onto a Jaguar E-Type V12, and its accompanying owner, a man called Alan. Her mood had once again started to swing and this meant frequent changes in most things in her life including her partners; so, when she quickly became bored with Alan she started seeing a lovely guy called Ron. Ron uniquely didn't have smart car and I remember him as being really funny. Of all of my mother's male friends that I met, I liked him the most. He seemed to make my mother happy and my grandparents were both keen on him. He liked football and he had a real caring side to him. He was from Crystal Palace in South London where he lived alone with his mother who he had looked after since his father had died when he was still a boy. Of all the „Uncles" I was introduced to by my mother he was the closest to someone I thought that I would have liked to actually be in a family with. My mother must have had similar thoughts since I remember going to look at some beautiful houses near Bagshot once with them both. But as things invariably went with my mother when she was so excitable, suddenly it was all change and nice guy Ron became yesterday's news when she met John, a man who she did go on to marry. Looking back, I think that Ron was probably fortunate to get out when he did. I never warmed to John, maybe because I had got on so well with Ron, but my mother must have seen something in this successful business man who lived in an exclusive property in the desirable area of Kingston-Upon-Thames (I wonder what it could have been?). My mother soon moved into John's house and ironically, she engaged Sylvia, my former foster mother as a cleaner. I am not sure if any professional or ethical boundaries were crossed here, perhaps it was simply a case of my mother returning a favour!

By then, aged around ten, I had become much more aware of my mother's frailties. Still living with my grandparents, now my legal guardians, I deliberately distanced myself as much as I could from her and her new married life. I must have had a good instinct, even back then, as I remember that shortly after they were married, they had a tremendous fight, in which my mother went for John with a carving knife and he took refuge in the upstairs bedroom which thankfully had a lock on the inside. Not deterred by this obstacle she went on to make substantial cuts and gougings on the door in an attempt to get to John and explain more clearly the exact nature of her grievance. At some point though, all must have been forgiven, if not forgotten, as my mother became pregnant and the happy newlyweds looked forwards to the arrival of their new baby. Alas, unlike in most fairy-tales there wasn't to be a happy ending to that story as sadly my mother had a miscarriage; although in reality the prospect of her bringing up a young baby during that phase of her life doesn't bear thinking about. Resilience not being my mother's strong suit, this episode finished her marriage and her relationship with John. Seemingly not being able to be without someone to look after her (and as you can see there were plenty of those; at my last count I had seen at least nine "Uncles" come and go), she went back to Alan, and then back to Ron, and then she met Les.

When I look back, there does seem to have been a downwards trend in the standing of the men in my mother's life, if they were measured by their professional and financial status. Now in her early 30's, no longer in her prime and with a track record to live down, she was a bit like an ageing premier league footballer who finds himself playing in the lower leagues in order to continue to get a game each week. My mother, who had dated celebrities and restauranteurs, company directors and chartered accountants was now going out with Les, a taxi driver (the human equivalent of Crewe Alexander, not quite in the lowest league but certainly towards the foot of the second division).[1] I liked Les, mainly because my mother was very happy with him; she seemed more relaxed in his company and I was very relieved that she was out of her marriage with John (as I assume he was as well after the knife incident). As part of my mother's divorce settlement from her 12-month marriage to John, she acquired a high-performance car called a Gordon Keeble. An unusual choice given that she couldn't drive, but maybe not so strange given her predilection for fast cars. I like to think mum asked for the car as she knew that I was very taken by its sleek lines as I had I often sat in it and pretended

---

[1] To be clear, I am not making any personal comment on my mum's boyfriends based on their professional status or wealth, nor am I making any wider comment on the quality of a person in relation to their job role. I am simply highlighting how things had changed for my mother, who had always appeared to put a high value on wealth, status and the accompanying trappings when choosing her boyfriend's when she was younger.

to drive it in John's showroom. At some point soon after they met, Les crashed and wrote off his own taxi, and mum used to let him use the Gordon Keeble for his work; he must have been driving the most stylish taxi in town.

Following what had become a fairly predictable pattern, at the beginning of my mother's relationship with Les, things were fantastic and I started spending most weekends with her and Les' family. I quickly befriended Mark, Les' middle child, who was then aged 14, the closest in age to me. Everything was once again rosy; my mother liked Les very much and he adored her, was devoted to her, and would do anything for her (a prerequisite if you wanted to be my mother's partner). She was once again working in Selfridges and going through a period of relative stability. It was against this backdrop that I became increasingly under the spell and influence of Mark, Les' son who was about to give me the benefit of his experience of living life in the fast lane as he set about teaching me, his 12 year old apprentice, all the good and all the bad, that I needed to know.

From Les' house in a pretty residential area of Cheam, I quickly became familiar with the public transport system of the London Borough of Sutton as I accompanied Mark on his nefarious adventures. Initially I had liked Mark very much and looked up to him; in part because of his two years seniority but also because he appeared so exciting and experienced in the ways of the world compared to me. On our first outing we went to Battersea Fun Fair. Mark had somehow got hold of a £10 note (a colossal amount of money for two young boys in those days) and he generously paid for me to go on all the rides and games; including the shooting range where I turned out to be something of a crack shot. Three hits from three shots meant that we accumulated points and prizes all night, and Mark, seeing that he was backing a winner, kept the money coming. By the end of the evening, we were weighed down with our booty, of dubious quality and negligible value to be sure, but as precious to us two teenagers as the treasures from Aladdin's cave.

I was sated with my incredible haul and ready for home, but for Mark, older than me and advanced for his age, the evening was still incomplete. He required a touch of romance to make his night perfect and that meant he needed to meet a girl. Mark's MO of persistence and insistence as well as a thick skin when it came to rejection paid off and before long he found a girl who was willing to accompany him on the ghost train, on the condition that he paid of course, and off they went. Later, on our way home, Mark took great delight in bragging to me that whilst on the ghost train he had managed to finger this young lovely, ensuring that a good night was had by all. Mark had got his romance, his reward being a fistful of fanny; and I had got to be Wild Bill Hickock, my reward being an armful of fluffy toys. I like to think that perhaps Mark's conquest was given 50p for a bag of chips or one of the various dayglo prizes we had acquired from the shooting range as a lasting memory of the evening, but that seems unlikely. Too young to understand or really be impressed by the magnitude of Mark's triumph, I listened politely as we rode home on the top deck back to Cheam, thinking that my friendship with Mark had got off to an excellent start. I didn't realise at the time that I had unwittingly entered into some kind of Faustian Pact and the riches that flowed as a result of his friendship would be paid for by the temporary loss of my own moral compass.

Following in the footsteps of Charles Dickens' The Artful Dodger with me as Oliver Twist, Mark was about to introduce me to the time-honoured art of shop lifting; a past-time I was familiar with from friends in Frimley Green, but one that I had solemnly vowed I was never going to participate in. However, my resistance quickly dissolved under Marks tutelage. At first,

I felt guilty, but this soon stopped, and I just went with the flow and ran with the gang. As long as you weren't caught it was all good fun. On one occasion close to Bonfire Night, we were doing penny for the guy outside Marks and Spencer in North Cheam. Every so often we would take a break from our shambolic effigy of Guido Fawkes by nipping into the store and stealing sweets and chocolate to relieve the boredom. Once Mark even stole a toy for me from Selfridges when we were visiting my mother. When not out "nicking" from shops in London, I would play the pin ball machines in a cafe back in Frimley Green. I would also do this on the machines in North Cheam but with the added frisson of stealing empty bottles from the back of the off license and returning them to the front of the shop in order to claim the refund on the bottles. Like a distorted version of the economic model of the circular flow of income, we then of course spent this money on the machines again. With this near limitless supply of coins to play the "flippers" as you might Imagine, we all became pinball wizards.

Another pleasurable past-time which Mark introduced me to was playing pitch and putt golf at the local New Malden golf course. You hired a putter and a pitching club, played a shortened nine-hole course and then returned your clubs. I am sure the eagle eyed amongst you will have spotted the flaw in the owner's business model; Mark certainly did. After having had a most enjoyable time playing several rounds, Mark decided that we should pilfer the clubs, which we duly did by stashing one club down each trouser leg and then running straight legged through the bushes to the bus stop and our journey home. Of course, our plan likewise suffered from a fatal flaw; since having illegally acquired the clubs we could never return to the club and we were never able to play again the game we had so much enjoyed. Perhaps we didn't think that one through thoroughly enough, as this put an immediate halt to this pleasurable pastime for us and WTF were we going to do with four golf clubs and no golf course to play on anyway! I was fast realising that perhaps Mark was not the criminal master mind I had at first taken him to be.

By now the honeymoon period between Mark and myself was over and our friendship began to turn sour. Mark could be extremely aggressive and he would often lose his temper and threaten me and bully me to do things I didn't want to. For a while I tolerated this and we continued to hang out together. Until Mark forced my involvement in his next criminal caper, one in which he had considerably upped the ante with a plan to break into his next-door neighbour's house. Our, or more accurately my, access being via one back garden to the other. Mark was not a complete criminal novice and he had judged that this high-risk job needed more serious planning and reconnaissance than usual, and therefore I had to climb up the high wooden fence that separated the two properties to case the joint first. During this trial run as I balanced precariously 10 foot in the air on the narrow ledge, Mark came running up frantically shouting and warning me that there was somebody coming. My novice cat burglar's nerves and reflexes were not up to this and in a panic, I attempted to descend too quickly and fell, landing with my full weight on my arm and instantly breaking it. Returning to school the story behind my broken arm was tricky to explain and had to be managed carefully for obvious reasons, not least Mark's predictably violent response if the real reason behind my injury ever got back to his father. So instead, I concocted a story that I had done it at the fairground on the rocket ride and I maintained this fiction for several years afterwards.

I was beginning to conclude that Mark's influence on me was neither well intentioned or positive, and in all likelihood, if nothing changed, would go on to get me into serious trouble.

Whether this was my own emerging moral conscience, or more a result of a recent shoplifting scare when I had been caught and given an almighty bollocking by a shopkeeper in Cheam and threatened with the Police I don't know; I would like to think it was the former but suspect it was the latter. But by now I had finally got wise to Mark and I pledged to myself that I would give up my life of crime and go straight.

About the same time, I was also beginning to develop more confidence in myself and had awakened to the realisation that above all else Mark was a bully, and he relied on this intimidation to maintain his power over me. A few months after my accident, together with some friends, I had started taking karate classes and had become good friends with some of the tougher, football playing kids at school. And in our efforts to emulate our hero, Bruce Lee, from the King Fu films, we constantly play sparred with each other and I got used to throwing and receiving punches and kicks in these good-natured battles. In addition to this, only a few weeks previously I had witnessed an event which turned out to be something of a humiliation for Mark and one after which he immediately seemed less invincible and threatening. Mark, myself and my cousin Jeffery had all gone together to the cinema. Inside the cinema Jeffrey got into an argument with a boy whilst we were buying ice creams and Mark sucker punched (a shameful tactic in which you punch someone often from behind and without warning) the boy when he wasn't looking. After the film when we were leaving the cinema, the boy was waiting for Mark. Mark picked up a brick and threatened the boy with it, but the boy did not run away and catching Mark off guard he punched him hard in the face. Mark started crying and was made to eat humble pie and I remember secretly feeling pleased that he had got his just desserts. Somehow armed with my emerging new confidence, my new combat skills, and the memory of Mark being beaten up at the cinema, Mark now seemed less scary and threatening, and I was determined and far better equipped to deal head on with his constant aggressive outbursts. By then I was determined that enough was enough and I knew that I had to make a stand against Mark.

My mother's relationship with Les was now also waning and her health was cycling downwards once again. Perhaps I sensed that I had less investment in the ongoing relationship with Les' family, but things had altered and so had my attitude towards Mark. I do not remember the specific bullying incident from Mark that caused my stand, but I do remember shouting at him that I was no longer afraid of him. If he wanted to try and hurt me, he could, but that I wasn't going to give in, and that whatever happened, I was going to explain everything to my mother. I think it was my final threat that deterred him most as more than anything he feared the ensuing consequences from his father. Shortly afterwards my mother left Les and returned to Ron, and then Alan, and then back to Ron again, that's how it went, perhaps most significantly for me I had got away from Mark's negative and potentially disastrous influence.

Parties

As a kid, I loved going to parties and there were always lots of them to go to. Most of my schoolfriends threw parties when it was their birthday (for obvious domestic reasons I never did) and being reasonably popular I received a lot of invites. As we got older these parties provided an opportunity for us boys to continue with our experimentation and curiosity in getting to know a bit more about girls. I guess I was fortunate in that being part of the in crowd, comparatively wholesome and not unattractive; girls quite liked me. Boys and girls used to "fancy each other" back in those days, and there were certainly a number of girls who I fancied the pants off (for me back then that was just an expression although it took on a different meaning as I got older). Very often at these parties we would play Spin the Bottle, the rules of which were very simple. We all sat round in a circle with a glass bottle in the middle, the person whose turn it was spun the bottle and had to kiss whoever it faced when it stopped spinning. In those unenlightened days if the bottle ended up pointing to someone of the same sex you respun (or at least you did at the parties I went to) it would have added a whole new dimension to the game had we not applied that rule. The wonderful simplicity of this game being that the more times you spun, the bottle the more girls you got to kiss. The randomness and immediacy of this game was perfect for me, particularly because my confidence and communication skills lagged way behind my physical desires. This simple game of chance avoided me having to go through the painful ritual of approaching and talking to a girl before any petting took place, and in just one evening I could get to kiss all the girls I spent so much time fantasising about - Aaah such innocent fun. After playing this teenage version of speed dating with the job done (yes, simple kissing was the ultimate goal in those early days), the boys would then march outside and have a game of football a new-found spring in our steps and sparkle in our eyes (God knows what the girls did).

No school year was complete at St Tar's without the annual treading of the boards in our school play. These events were a magical experience from the start: the auditions, the casting, the rehearsals, the set design, trying out your costumes and then taking them home to be modified, and of course finally the nights of the big show. We always seemed to do three nights and I am sure, as with most school and Am Dram productions, of the three shows, one was always crap where everything went wrong, one was alright, and one was brilliant.

It couldn't have been further away from the West End or Broadway if it tried, but the feelings of excitement and exhilaration, once everyone was transformed by their costumes and make up and the lights dimmed and the curtains opened, could not have been beaten. I am absolutely certain it cannot have been anything like as much fun on the other side of the stage as it was for us players, and had we been a bit less high we might have observed this in the expressions on the faces of the audience as they sat through an hour and a half of yet another school interpretation of Aladdin.

These and similar public events at school brought with them their own inherent risks in that they were occasions when my grandparents would cross the divide into my school life with some inevitable exposure to my peers and/or their families. My fragile ego was overly concerned that their presence in loco parentis graphically represented my home life to the outside world (apart from the times when my mum turned up accompanied by her latest beau in a fancy sports car) so different than that of my friends. Although I hated the times when these two worlds collided, looking back I recall that they could produce occasions of humour, certainly far funnier than anything taking place on the stage. One year we performed Ali Baba and the 40 Thieves; and in this production I had a minor part as one of the thieves. My lasting memory is from the night my grandparents came to watch. While I was off stage my grandfather, needing to relieve himself, and having lived his lifetime in the African bush, simply walked outside and around to the back of the hall to do his business. I can still feel my cheeks flushing with embarrassment as one of the cast shouted "oh look, there's an old guy out there having a slash," and when I turned to look, of course it was my grandad urinating against the fence at the back of the building. I never said anything at the time to hide my shame, but as I reflect now with the added benefit of the passing of time, I remember this moment with great fondness and I often wonder what this displaced old man was thinking. Despite all his difficulties, he and my grandmother had taken me on when my mother wouldn't or couldn't, and they both loved me deeply in their own ways. I like to think that if I had my time again, I would call out to him as he let forth his stream "Hey dad, enjoy your piss, take your time you're not missing anything". Nobody ever knew that it was my grandad having a pee and to be fair, as self-absorbed as we all were at the time, nobody was really that interested either.

Around 1975, one of the most important influences in my life was going to emerge from a most unlikely direction. Father Bernard Rowley the new Catholic priest for the parish of Frimley visited St Tar's with the Canadian number one ranked women's table tennis player (relax everyone this is one of the good stories about catholic priests from the 1970's). Father Rowley, as well as being a priest, was also a two-star table tennis coach and quite influential in the English Table Tennis Association, and he wanted to develop a table tennis school of excellence which would provide a sporting focus for many of the children in his new parish. The nuns who were by now running our school were delighted to welcome Father Rowley to the school to put on an exhibition match with the female Champion. It was a fantastic display as Father Rowley could be a bit of a show off (he once beat my friend Keith, who had been playing for a few years, playing with a biscuit tin lid). The result was that several pupils, including myself, joined his training program and a number of us signed up to join the Frimley Table Tennis Club as juniors; this led to my next major involvement and for a while, obsession in a new sport.

Playing table tennis became a passion for me. I spent thousands of hours practicing and being coached by Father Rowley along with many other youngsters. I made some really good new friends through table tennis; people who seemed to take a genuine interest in me for myself rather than my ability to commit petty burglary. I am truly grateful to Father Rowley for the time, commitment and financial investment he put into us kids. I did show some aptitude for the game and I trained incredibly hard, having by then given up playing football and lost a lot of interest in karate. I think that Father Rowley recognised my potential and was also aware of my home life situation, but I don't think I ever really fulfilled these ambitions; although I had the commitment and some talent, I was never as naturally gifted as you needed to be to progress much beyond the junior county level.

I loved playing table tennis, it certainly kept me fit as I took the training part very seriously, but also it provided a structure and a distraction for me at a time in my life when I needed it most. Many years later Father Rowley confided to me that he had seen playing table tennis as a way for me to take my mind off the traumas and problems in my home life and my mother. He was pretty canny and caring, and I was sorry to read that he had died suddenly in October 2006.

Chapter 5 - Growing up

During the time I was at St Tarcisius it changed from being an infant and junior school to being a middle school. The main impact of this for the majority of the pupils was that instead of transferring to secondary school at age 11 we transferred at age 13 i.e. in old money the third year of secondary education but now known as year 9. Several of my friends at the time, including Tom Bartlett, had elected to sit the 11+ exam. Success in this was and still is (where they exist) the selection process for these children to progress out of the cattle herd of a comprehensive education and into a grammar school. In our case these bright kids went onto the local Catholic grammar school, Salesian College in Farnborough. Although by that time I was doing very well at school and was in most of the top sets, I felt anxious and intimidated by this prospect and did not want to sit the 11+, preferring instead to stay with the majority of my friends and transfer to the main catholic secondary school in our area, St John the Baptist (SJB) in Old Woking (perhaps the most famous ex pupil being Sean Lock the comedian who sadly died in 2021). On starting at St Johns, I was determined to do well and worked even harder at my studies making good progress academically. I was very conscious of the step up in the amount of homework demanded of us and I endeavoured to do as much of it as possible on the school bus on the way to and from school so that I could have more time to devote to training and playing table tennis matches.

A major consequence of commencing our secondary education one year later than everyone else was that we started studying our GCSE subjects one year later as well. Almost as soon as we had begun at St John's we had to start thinking about which subjects we wanted to take at GCSE. This process of selecting your subjects was known as "making your options" and looking back seems inherently unfair and educationally unsound even, given that we had so little chance to properly experience the wider curriculum subjects before having to select those we wished to study for the next two years[2]. My natural academic talents lay in maths and the sciences (particularly physics and chemistry) so these were an obvious choice and to these I added German, photography and business studies. English language and English literature were compulsory but unfortunately not my strong suit, particularly the latter. I worked hard and did well, but my analytical skills far outweighed my communication skills; whereas I was ranked at the top of the year in maths and science, I was way down in English.

I continued to play football for the school, but this was becoming increasingly more competitive with a much larger pool of players to choose from and my place in the school team was no longer a foregone conclusion. But between my football, ongoing karate and table tennis matches, I was becoming incredibly fit; I was running about two miles every morning before school to supplement my table-tennis training. I was progressing though the Aldershot league table tennis divisions and was playing in Frimley's A team in the first division. I was also being groomed for the Under 17 County Leagues as well, largely thanks to Father Rowley's strong links with the Sussex table-tennis leagues. I lived, breathed and ate table tennis for a while. I was travelling all around the country to play in tournaments, and if I wasn't playing table-tennis I was watching it. Father Rowley used to drive several of us enthusiasts to

---

[2] This narrowing down was important as far as your future career and life choices were concerned and a continuing aspect of our education system seem s to be to specialise from an early stage. You narrowed down for GCSE (O-level) choices and then narrowed down again two years later for GCSE A-level subject; which to a large extent determines what degree courses are available to you should you go down a more traditional higher education route.

Birmingham and Brighton to watch the National and European Championships, which was a phenomenal motivator for a young fan to be able to watch close up some of the world's best players at that time.

These trips to tournaments were accompanied with the additional excitement of Father Rowley's driving. Somewhere in Father Rowley's family connections (I think it was his brother) he must have had some other source of private income as he always owned very expensive, large, fast cars. I remember a Wolseley 2.2 litre and then a Rover 3500 SD1, which boasted a top speed of 125mph. Father Rowley loved to drive these beasts at breakneck speed on the straights and into the curves. We kids sitting in the back were both exhilarated and terrified at the same time, grinning hysterically at each other as we overtook car after car, often on what seemed like blind bends. Whether it was Father Rowley's driving skills or Divine intervention we fortunately avoided accidents and furthermore Father Rowley was never stopped by the Police for speeding. Maybe they couldn't catch him, or perhaps he was being looked after from above. We always seemed to arrive just in time, regardless of how late we set off or what traffic we encountered, shaking slightly and thankful that we lived to tell the tale once again.

My mum's decline

Around the time I started at St John's I had begun to see far less of my mother as my studies, sport and my emerging social life filled most of my time. I no longer visited any of the places my mother lived at, partly as by then she had become much more transient and her accommodation arrangements were often quite temporary. For a while she returned to stay with my grandparents and me in Frimley Green and she got a job locally as a secretary. It was during this period that we frequently went to the cinema since she was, and I was to become, a big movie fan. She liked action films and I vividly remember going to see some of the blockbusters of the day with her, including, Jaws, the Street Fighter, and Every Which Way but Loose. These are fond and poignant memories, and there is no doubt looking back that by then my mother was in seriously declining mental health. One of her big heroes was Muhammed Ali, and we loved to watch boxing together on the TV; I think she had known one or two prize-fighters during the peak of her London social life. I remember her shouting and cheering jubilantly as we listened on the radio to Ali's Rumble in the Jungle fight with the World Champion George Foreman. She was elated as Ali used his genius "rope a dope" tactics for the first time to tire out Foreman and win by a knock out in the eighth round. To this day I still thoroughly enjoy a good movie, more often than not in a comfy armchair together with my wife and/or two boys, and I still love the thrill of a good prize-fight, although I don't think I have ever seen anyone fight with the same combination of intelligence, artistry and skill that Ali showed at his peak.

Something else which I have to thank my mother for, is that she introduced me to the game of chess when I was about six or seven. Although both of us were unskilled at the game, we spent a lot of close hours in combat with each other. I grew to love that game and one benchmark of my growing skill was that I got good enough to beat Tom Bartlett. This was the only mental challenge in which I could beat Tom as he surpassed me in all other areas. I am really grateful to my mother for this introduction as I still love and play chess (online now with people from all over the world), and on balance I win as many as I lose. It has helped me keep my mind sharp particularly at times of great stress and during periods of depression.

I mentioned earlier that by the end of my first year at SJB (year 9) during the Summer months I was running about two miles each day as part of my school journey. On one occasion I arrived home to find that nobody was in. This was not unusual and so I turned on the TV and got something to eat from the fridge. Thinking about the empty house situation a bit longer, I reasoned that my mother should be in, and I thought she was probably having a nap upstairs as she did have a tendency to sleep a lot, particularly when she was depressed. After watching a bit more TV and by then having finished my snack I went upstairs to see how she was, and I found her not sleeping but unconscious on her bed having overdosed from a bottle of tablets, which was still sitting on the table next to the bed. It cannot have been a major overdose as I was able to rouse her and bring her some tea until eventually my grandmother came home and took over. This was not my mother's first overdose and on reflection it seemed unlikely that it was a serious suicide attempt given the low number of tablets she appeared to have taken. By now, as I was older and more emotionally perceptive, I began to appreciate the severity of my mother's mental ill health and how her depression could come down on her at any time, triggered by the slightest of reasons. I believe that from then onwards my self-preservation instincts kicked in and I started building a stronger mental wall by shutting out some of my feelings of love and dependency on my mother. My 13-year-old ego had determined my mother's behaviour to be an act of selfishness and I was not going to be sympathetic towards her continued self-destruction. I rationalised this as being my adolescent way of coping, my instinct for survival helping me to manage a situation that had become too painful for me to bear and enabling me to cope with events that were completely off track and outside of my control.

A few weeks before my mother eventually killed herself, I had gone with her to meet her new boyfriend, Bob, at his home. My mum wanted to introduce me to him so that the two of us could get to know each other. Bob, another taxi driver, was a portly middle-aged guy with a prominent moustache. I remember comparing him unfavourably with some of her previous boyfriends thinking that she really was playing in the lower divisions now. I never really got to know Bob or anything much about him, apart from I knew that he carried a gun in the glove compartment in his taxi. He had proudly showed this to me one day saying that it was for "in case things ever turn nasty". I saw Bob very rarely and when I did it was mainly when he came to my grandparent's house, either to pick up or to drop off my mother. I deliberately took little interest in him or their life together since I had started rationalising my mother's life as being something separate from my own; it just felt easier that way given that she was such an inconsistent and unreliable feature, flitting in and out of my world, more often than not accompanied by scenes of high drama. I think my mother also sensed this and knew that our relationship was becoming more distant. Of course, I still loved her a lot and looked forward to seeing her and spending time together, but she had somehow become an extra in my life. I had schooled myself so that I was no longer dependent upon our relationship or her love, and I no longer got upset when she went away again.

The last time I saw my mother had been on a visit to Bob's. Bob lived in a big house in Godalming, where he had converted the top floor to rent out to lodgers. At that time, he had three young graduates from British Aerospace living there, who I found a lot more entertaining and interesting than boring, fat Bob. I remember my mother being on good form that day, she joked around with the three guys and myself and brought us sandwiches and tea on a tray. On the way home in the car, she casually asked me if I might like to come and live with her and Bob at his home. I flatly refused to this throwing something of a tantrum. I argued that my whole life, my school, my friends, my football team were all in Frimley Green and nothing could or would make me move. I was very conscious of Bob sitting in the driver's seat, with his shooter locked and loaded just inches away, saying nothing. Maybe he was relieved thinking that this was a good result, as he wouldn't have one more mouth to feed after all. Perhaps he even imagined that he had dodged a bullet on this occasion when things had indeed "turned nasty". But this is of course purely conjecture on my part, based on my prejudicial feelings towards him at the time and the accompanying threats that his relationship with my mother posed to my settled existence. Bob had never been unkind or unfriendly towards me. It is perhaps actually more likely that he had been genuinely pleased to extend his generous offer of welcoming me into his home if it was my mother's desire, and if it meant that she would be happier, more settled and he could keep her close to him. I'll never know. I do know that my veto pretty much ended the subject and something of a silence descended for the remainder of the journey. I said thank you to Bob and gave my mum a goodbye hug and a kiss not realising at the time that this was to be the last time I would ever see her.

The following weekend I was staying in Aldershot at my Auntie Myra's, with Julie and Chris. On the Saturday morning I heard a knocking on the front door followed by my Uncle Vernon's voice. This was an unusual event in itself as Myra and Vernon having separated somewhat acrimoniously some years previously had very little to do with each other. From where I was sleeping, I could hear that Vernon sounded upset as he apologised to Myra explaining that he urgently needed to see me. He came into my room and struggling to keep his emotions under control, told me that my mother was dead. I was devastated to hear this and wept and sobbed for a long time. I wept for my mother, I wept for myself, and I wept because of the physical pain and emptiness that had descended into the pit of my stomach. I think part of me had been readying myself for this moment following my mum's previous attempts of overdosing, cutting her wrists and unsuccessful hanging, but nothing could have prepared me for this earth-shattering news. Only minutes before I had been fast asleep enjoying my teenage dreams and then I had suddenly been awakened into every child's worst nightmare.

After regaining some control of myself, I got dressed and Vernon took me back to my grandparents. Although my mother and Vernon had not spent a whole lot of time with each other in recent years, they had been very close, and Vernon was himself in deep shock and distress over the death of his younger sister. Through his tears he explained that he had received a phone call from Bob that morning. Bob had told him that he come back after a night's taxi shift and had found my mother dead, hanging from a belt she had placed around her neck, inside a large wardrobe. In the car with Vernon, I found myself hating her and blaming her for carrying out such a selfish act and leaving me on my own. I had by that time long since stopped looking to my mother for love and my wellbeing. As I had been seeing her less frequently, she had begun to feel more like a special auntie than a mother. Someone who arrived unexpectedly and unannounced with gifts and wonderful things for me to do, and less like a parent who would keep me safe and secure. When we were together, she always tried to give me her full attention and she attempted to be happy and in good spirits for my benefit; even though I could see that she was struggling. But in that exact moment as my world reeled around, I was too overwhelmed by my own loss and heartbreak to acknowledge this.

It is poignantly significant to me that the coroner's verdict on my mother's death was "death by misadventure" - rather than death by suicide. This ruling is not uncommon where the dead person had previously been mentally ill as evidenced by regular and recent involvement with psychiatric services. In my mother's case I hypothesise that the coroner judged her as being acutely unwell before her death, "not of sound mind" and therefore not fully aware or responsible for the consequences of her own actions i.e., the full implications of taking her own life. Over time I would come to sympathise with and share the State's more considered and sympathetic interpretation on my mother's death based on her mental health, but at the time my overriding emotions of hurt and abandonment resulted in my less charitable judgement. [3]

Soon after my mother's suicide I began to experience my first feelings of anxiety as my teenage brain dwelt on her death and I began to obsess over the fact that my grandparents, then aged 65 and 70, were my only direct remaining family now. Alone in bed at night I worried about what would become of me if something happened to them. I found these constant thoughts of death and my own future so terrifying that I could not face the trauma of going to my mother's funeral. I just wasn't ready to face the absolute reality of her death and now that I had managed to stem my tears, I didn't want to find myself breaking down again in front of all the concerned well-wishers. And so, I didn't attend the funeral ceremony and cremation at Aldershot crematorium. It wasn't until many years later when I attended my grandmother's funeral, and I visited the chapel where my mother's service was held that I finally said my goodbyes in person to her.

On the evening of my mother's funeral, my grandfather was in the kitchen whilst I was in the front room watching TV, and I

---

[3] Changes to the law in 2018, have resulted in coroners being given more latitude in ruling suicide if they judge it probable that the actions taken by the individual which caused their own death were deliberate and that it is probable that they intended to cause their own death through these actions.

heard him coughing repeatedly. I shouted through to him, but he didn't reply, and I could hear that his coughing had got louder and more frantic. When I went to see how we was, he was bent double with his hands on his knees; his face had turned purple and just as I moved towards him, he toppled onto the floor in a faint. Thankfully he came around almost immediately and appeared OK, incurring just a bruise on his head; he went on to have several similar attacks over the next few years. This event did nothing to alleviate my concerns over my grandparent's mortality and my own future. After a while in the house things did return to some kind of normality, and my grandmother soon resumed her shouting at my grandfather and complaining that he hadn't got off the sofa all day or done anything or changed his clothes (which he frequently slept in) for over a week. At least my Uncle Peter was back with us for a while; he was good company for my grandfather as together they relived memories of Africa and the very different lives, they both used to have. My mother was now dead and cremated, but outwardly little else had changed; at the end of the Christmas holiday, I returned to school along with everyone else and if anyone asked if I'd had a good holiday, I replied flatly that it had been okay and said nothing about my mother.

For the next few years life continued for me much as it had been, a combination of studying, playing sport and socialising, until finally the Summer of '81 arrived and all my hard studying at school was over; I had taken my A-levels and, subject to satisfactory results, I would be off to Kent University in the Autumn to study for a maths degree. It felt like this was the Summer my whole life had been leading up to; I was feeling good, my confidence was sky high and I felt invincible. My friend Tim and I both had Honda motorbikes; not the fastest or most stylish bikes on the road but renowned for their quality and reliability, and we went on countless trips together during the warm weather. Added to that Keith had passed his driving test and had reasonable access to his dad's car and the 3 of us spent a lot of time together touring the local village pubs. Fortunately I was earning some money working as a painter and decorator on a job that my friend Mark Ojay had got for me at GQ Defence. We frequently worked outdoors, which suited me fine as it meant I could also work on my tan (something I had become a bit obsessive about in my late teens). I was working with Mark on the day our exam results came through and it had been a bit awkward as he hadn't done very well and was going to have to do resits, whereas I had got all the grades I needed; and nothing now could stop me going to Kent. Somewhat ironically, I ran into Mark a few years later at a time when life had become very tough for me: Mark was by then established in a well-paid career as a computer programmer and about to get married. I was pleased for him. Not least because he had been a good friend and a nice bloke.

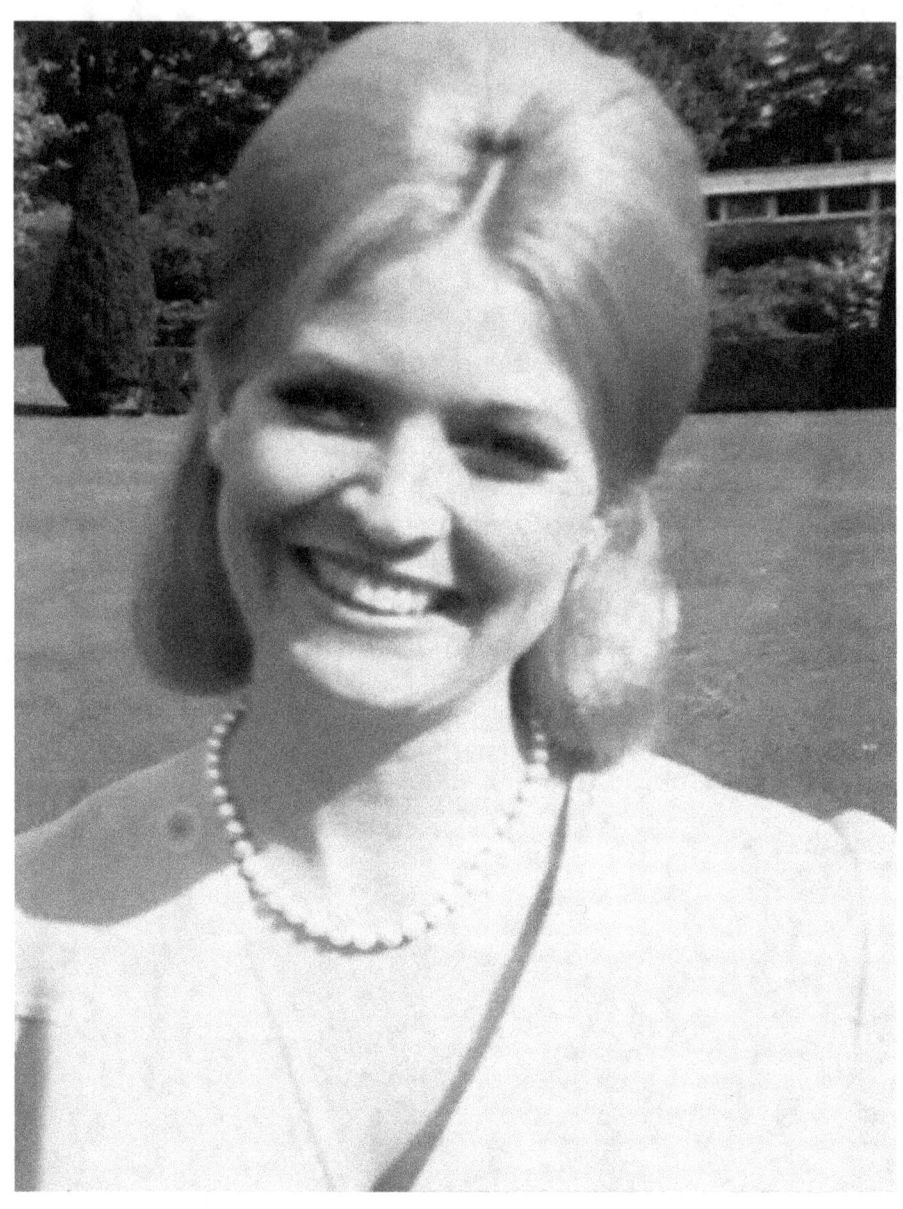

<u>Mum not long before she died.</u>

Chapter 6 - End of the line

The wheels fall off the bus - Kent University, October 1981 to November 1981

Did I say I was riding high at the beginning of Summer 81? Well, pride comes before a fall. I am not sure if Isaac Newton was the first person to coin the phrase "what goes up must come down," but unbeknownst to me I was about to get a front seat in this lesson on life. Having achieved my required A-level grades I set off to Kent University, situated in the historic City of Canterbury, to study for a degree in maths. Kent was and still is a very good university and there was no doubting that I had done well. At first, I had a ball as a fresher, partying and meeting lots of interesting people. A whole new social world was being unveiled to me, the lectures hadn't even started yet and I was already on a journey that was expanding my horizons through meeting new people from new backgrounds with new ideas. I was being bombarded every day by new geography, new sounds, new sights; everything was new, new, new. After only a few days however, I began to feel a bit overwhelmed as I struggled to absorb and assimilate this constant flood of new experiences which had begun to feel like an assault on my senses. Although at the time I was unaware of my inherited illness, it seems likely looking back that I was fast approaching the end of a high/manic phase in my bipolar condition and the pattern of what was about to come next was almost inevitable.

Life had certainly been full throttle over the previous year with my studies, social life, and the glorious summer I had just enjoyed. I was making friends at university easily and was already part of an established social group of people. Whilst I was socialising and having fun in their company, I found I could push my emerging feelings of anxiety away and ignore them for a while. My real difficulties began to emerge when my course started properly and the actual learning commenced, in theory at least. At school I had always excelled at maths, it came easily to me and I was pretty much always the top of the class, but now, for the first time in my life, I could not make sense of any of the concepts or theories that were being taught in the lectures and tutorials or in the books we were told to read. This should not have been the case; I had earned and demonstrated my credentials to be on the course through achieving good grades in my A-levels. And yet, everything was confusing, I just couldn't get it no matter how long I stared blankly at the attempts at notes I took in the lectures. The maths felt completely beyond me and I was totally out of my depth and alone with this knowledge. Rather than seek help or speak to a tutor at this early stage (which might have proved useful in easing some of the pressure) I chose the alternative route of distraction and pushing the problem down deep inside me as I continued to lead a very active social life, learning about music, discussing politics and engaging in interesting debates with the other new students. This was of course a naive and foolish strategy and everyday my anxiety grew, increasingly gnawing away at the back of my mind until I could feel myself losing control and feared that already my dreams were slipping away.

Each morning I would awake after a restless night's sleep, feeling totally unrefreshed as if I had not slept at all. I was physically drained from the moment I started my day. This exhaustion weighed me down further throughout the afternoon and my lectures. Somehow for a while it seemed that I was able to reinvigorate myself by the time the evening arrived; on an artificial high I would launch myself back into my social life, but underneath I knew my bravado was false, my foundations were unstable to say the least, and little by little I was falling apart. The next day would begin again with the familiar feelings of despair, dragging my mind and body through another unbearable day of incomprehension and futility; I was just going through the motions because I didn't know what else to do. I kept taking endless notes during the lectures in the vain hope that if I could only find time and space and the right frame of mind, things might fall into place and it would all become clear to me; of course it never did. My notes might just as well have been written in double Dutch as the theorems and concepts they represented remained indecipherable to me. And so, in November to protect any remaining sanity and self-esteem I had left, I dropped out from University less than two months after my anticipated life changing career had started. Somehow at the time I rationalised this decision to myself as necessary to protect any future opportunity at Higher Education (HE). I told the university and anyone else that cared enough to listen that I had had enough of university and I just wanted to get a job. It seems hilarious to me now that that was the line I spun; implying that there were better things waiting for me in the world of manual and menial employment on minimum wages. Still, I don't suppose anyone believed that bullshit, I certainly didn't; but even the mentally ill have to try and retain some self-respect.

The worst Christmas for a long time

So, two short months after leaving home, I was back in Frimley Green with my grandparents in the middle of a cold, damp and gloomy November; my academic ambitions torn to shreds and my self-esteem on the floor. To be honest, at the time I was grateful to at least be somewhere familiar where I hoped I could hide and rest up, recover my energy and attempt to avoid a total mental collapse - it turned out I had no idea. I thought I was depressed at University, but my spirits were to plummet even further after I got home, when the full significance of what had happened sunk in, and dark thoughts about my future filled my every spare moment (of which I had plenty). For the first time I wondered if there was something fundamentally wrong with me and I empathised with the despair that my mother must have felt and why she had eventually chosen to end her life.

At the time I had not got a name for my condition and I had never been to the doctors to discuss my emotional wellbeing. Despite my mother's history and what I had seen of her illness the whole world of mental health and the different conditions, including bipolar, was completely unknown to me. All I knew was how I felt. Only a few months before I was elated and on top of the world but now I felt physically and emotionally exhausted, depressed and worthless. I had witnessed similar patterns in my mother, who constantly careened between precariously animated and volatile high energy periods to the depths and destructive anxieties that accompanied her severe lows, which followed on as predictably as night follows day. The consequence of which were her repeated breakdowns, overdoses and suicide attempts, which she experienced from her teenage years onwards. I began to consider more closely the characters of my grandmother and my grandfather and believed I could see some of the inherited qualities that dominated my mother's character and I then began to see some similarities with my own feelings and behaviours (and of course God knows what emotional frailties my father's genes may have brought to the party). Although I don't remember too much about medical interventions during this first low period for me, I do know that I did start taking anti-depressants for the first time; initially they didn't seem to do anything but I persevered and as the winter months wore on, I gradually started to feel a little better. This improvement in my state of mind was, if not exclusively down to the pharmacological interventions, certainly helped by them and now some 40 years later, I am still taking daily medication to keep my mental health in balance.

My gap year

During the early months of 1982, I slowly pulled myself back from the brink of disaster and I was able to begin to look more objectively about my situation and my future. After all, lots of people drop out of university all the time and it wasn't the end of the world. I had regained a sufficient amount of my confidence and energy and I had begun to convince myself that I had overcome the depression that had caused my disastrous experience in Kent. In reality, my illness had probably reached the bottom of its cycle at that point and together with the help of the anti-depressants I was on an upward trajectory again. I say this because since recovering my energy and coming out of the depression I was now holding down three different part-time jobs simultaneously: one was working in a bar at the Working Man's Club in Camberley, the second was assembling motorbikes at Motorcycle City in North Camp, and the third was working at the weekends as a cashier at a petrol station. Although all the jobs were relatively low-skilled and low-paid, the combination of the three jobs together meant that I was earning a reasonable amount of money.

The Motorcycle City job is worth mentioning in a bit more detail (and it will crop up again a bit later) as this job provided me with a way back into a social life as well as putting money in my pocket. My job was assembling the final parts of the motorbikes e.g. handlebars, front wheel, wiring to the headlamps etc, after the bikes were sold, to make them roadworthy and ready to go to the customer. Ironically the trickiest part of the job was often taking the motorbike out of the wooden frame it was delivered in. At first I was paid on piece rate of £3 a bike, and I enjoyed the fun and the banter with the other guys in the yard which was a constant accompaniment whilst we worked. I became something of a specialist in doing the more fiddly bikes that no one else wanted to do, and this meant that I was able to set up my own mini production line and finish three identical bikes in about an hour and a half, the net financial result to me being £9, about £25 an hour by today's standards. Not bad at the time for a 19 year old, particularly one who was only a few months past his first mental breakdown. I used to think the work I was doing was pretty unskilled and menial at the time but of course it was critically important to the new owner that their brakes would work properly and that the front wheel wasn't going to fall off, so it was probably a more responsible role than I appreciated at the time.

Between them, all three jobs kept me busy and provided a much-needed focus and a release for all the pent-up energy that was now coursing through my veins once again after having sat like a zombie in my grandparents' home for four months since I left Kent. Also, a very real and urgent financial crisis had arisen at home that threatened to take away the roof over my grandparents and my head. A problem which needed an immediate injection of cash to resolve and which in reality at that time could only come from me. Unbeknownst to me, some years earlier my Uncle Vernon, who had financial difficulties of his own, had borrowed money from a loan shark, which he had secured against my grandparents' house, and whilst I was away at university this loan had fallen due. Although I loved Vernon dearly, in retrospect he was always a financial disaster who constantly boasted (perhaps more for his own self esteem than anything else) that the big business deal that was going to make his fortune was just around the corner; but of course, it never materialised. By the early months of 1982 my grandparents could no longer keep hidden the threatening messages regularly arriving in the post as the foreclosure letters were coming in thick and fast. It was only by using my earnings to pay off the loan shark that the situation was resolved and the debt paid off. I am not really one to believe in Karma, but at times I have pondered over what would have happened if I hadn't dropped out of Kent University in 1981, because I certainly couldn't have paid off this debt had I still been there. Every cloud has a silver lining however and in the process of paying off this debt, and partly to prevent anything similar happening again, I insisted that my name was subsequently added to the title deeds of the house; thereby establishing me as the rightful owner in the event of my grandparents death. This was to prove a life saver for me in the future.

During the madness of Spring 1982 and the full-on distraction of holding down three jobs, I had gradually begun to feel a lot more positive and hopeful that my mental troubles were behind me and that everything would be okay going forwards; it was whilst in this buoyant resurgent mood that I had started to consider a second attempt at Higher Education. Once again, I was confident that I had the academic intellect required to study for a degree and I told myself that it was all about choosing the right subject and course for me. This time I lowered my sights in the HE hierarchy and turned my focus towards Polytechnics; since I was fairly sure that I had burned my bridges as far as a university place was concerned and also I thought that a more practical based, technical course might better suit me (after my Kent experience I was keen to stay clear of mind bending mathematical theorems and concepts which my brain couldn't cope with). So once more I found myself trawling through prospectuses and submitting multiple applications, this time to study computer science. I remember receiving an early rejection from Brighton Polytechnic, who I suspected had seen straight through me, but Thames Polytechnic were more amenable, accepting my explanation of a change of chosen career paths and they offered me a place commencing in October 1982.

The rest of 1982 leading up to my start at Polytechnic continued at a breakneck pace. I managed to pass my driving test and bought an old Triumph Spitfire sports car from a guy at Motorcycle City. I knew the car needed a lot of work doing on it but I completely overestimated my mechanical expertise as well as my perseverance for the task, and so I quickly passed the car on to Tim, who possessed these two attributes in spades and he soon got it running. Instead, I traded up my motorbike to a Yamaha SR500, having sold my Honda 250 to my lodger Shaun. At this point I should introduce Shaun a bit more fully as he does have some significance in my story. Shaun was also an assembler at Motorcycle City; I didn't really know him that well and perhaps not being the best judge of character, and also never able to turn down a financial opportunity, I offered him the chance to lodge at my grandparent's house. My calculated thinking was that this way I stood a greater chance of getting the remainder of the instalments that he still owed me for the motorbike and also that the £20 a week rent would be useful for my grandmother. I didn't ever really consider how my grandparents would view a complete stranger coming to live with us or even what the dynamics would be like of having another person living in our small house.

It is clear to me now, when I look back, that Shaun had his own issues. Initially he seemed a very nice guy but as the weeks wore on, he became increasingly disrespectful and aggressive towards me, constantly putting me down in front of others at work. Perhaps as a result of my Mark Dickmond experience, this was not new territory to me, and I had already learned an important lesson in how far I was willing to let things go before I said enough was enough. One day at work, Shaun made one too many snide comments at my expense, and so I turned and punched him. We had a small scuffle which spilled out from the showroom onto the street. Fortunately, my better physical condition and karate training meant that I came out on top; in fact, I don't think he landed a single blow on me "float like a butterfly sting like a bee" (that was me mum). Amazingly, neither of us was dismissed, and afterwards Shaun totally changed his attitude towards me and we became much better and more equal friends. This probably is not the best foundation for a friendship, but it almost certainly increased the likelihood of Shaun maintaining his bike repayments and paying his weekly rent. I think at heart Shaun was a decent chap and any concerns I had about him staying in my house when I went to polytechnic disappeared. Surprisingly to all of us, Shaun and my grandmother got on really well and he seemed to develop a bond of sorts with my grandfather, and the two of them frequently sat on the sofa, rolling their tobacco, watching TV together. Not sharing many words as they didn't have much in common to talk about, but weirdly in tune with each other.

In that Summer of '82, the sun was shining again and I felt fortunate to have fallen on my feet working with such a great gang of people. Whilst I was sure I would miss the crack of working at Motorcycle City, I was certain (in my euphoric state of mind) in my decision and I didn't have any space or time for doubts or second thoughts about my decision to go to polytechnic. I am not sure if it was prophetic, but I do remember one morning towards the end of Summer whilst in the middle of assembling a bike, I found myself staring to cry uncontrollably; similar to how I had cried when I was at Kent University. Although this was a bit shocking and disturbing, I dismissed it as being some kind of emotional release mechanism as I readied myself for my new life and I didn't think too much more about it. Fortunately, nobody in my group at Motorcycle City saw this or if they did no one said anything or asked me if I was okay; I wonder what might have poured forth if they had.

I firmly believed that at that time that I was closing down one chapter in my life and opening a new one as I made my final preparations to go off to polytechnic. I still had a couple of months to go before leaving and I chose to ease up on myself and reduce my workload to just working at Motorcycle City. I had learned from my previous experience and wanted to ensure that I started my studies in good mental and physical health (I still mistakenly thought I was in control of my emotions). At the end of September, I left Motorcycle City on good terms, and set off for Woolwich and take two.

Just pausing for a moment's reflection here. At this point in my life, I had been through what I hoped had been a singular episode of depression brought on by my inability to cope with my Kent University experience. I had been prescribed anti-depressants to help me though this low period and I believed that this one-off event was now behind me, as long as I took good care of myself. Certainly, no-one had mentioned or cautioned that I might have some kind of ongoing mental health condition that could reoccur, nor had any links been made to my mother's illness. At that time, diagnoses of bipolar were still very new and relatively rare, and I think that a wider approach of combination drug treatments for managing the condition was not yet common practice (I was on anti-depressants but nothing that might help manage any mood swings). Perhaps, even if anyone had been keeping an eye out for me, it would have been difficult to distinguish between what is the normal youthful exuberance and enthusiasm of a 19-year-old boy emerging after a major life setback, from the more worrying pattern of my cyclical mental ill health condition. But there were certainly some warning signs and red flags knocking about: a predisposition given my mother's long history and struggle with manic depression; the high leading up to my first breakdown at University, followed by the subsequent depression; and perhaps now again the hints from my behaviour that I might be cycling into another manic phase, holding down three jobs, the unrealistic ideas and actions I was taking, e.g. doing up a vintage sports car, and now these unexpected and unexplained emotional outbursts. Mind you if that's all it took, I am sure half the teenagers in the world could be diagnosed as bipolar.

Chapter 7 - Here comes the rain... again

The Thames Polytechnic episode

With the memories from what happened at Kent firmly in mind, my first priority when I started poly' was to be more measured from the outset in my socialising. I reckoned that if I took things more calmly this time round, I could remain in control. Everything started off well and unlike one year earlier, I found that I could follow and understand the lectures and information that was presented to us. I became friendly with a Scottish lad, James Cruickshank, who at the age of 23 was a mature student. James appeared a lot more experienced and worldly wise than me, having seen far more of life, including some time spent working on the boats in Scotland. We got on well, enjoying each other's sense of humour and taste in music. In this respect things were certainly different this time round; I was being far more moderate in my social life and I was coping academically. Sadly and ultimately tragically, other aspects of my previous experience at Kent soon started repeating themselves; if anything, even worse this time. Not long after starting at Poly', I began to feel more tired than anything I had ever experienced in my life before. I would go to bed and fall asleep relatively early, but when I woke up, I would still feel absolutely exhausted and fit for nothing other than crawling back into my bed. My unspoken private fears were becoming a reality and I could feel the black cloud of crippling depression descending over me once more. Exhaustion and debilitating fatigue are common symptoms experienced during bipolar depression, but it is not just feeling over tired; it can be an overwhelming lethargy that prevents the person suffering, from achieving even the simplest of tasks or stringing two thoughts together; indeed, this symptom can be helpful in establishing a diagnosis. My depression grew more intense and more absolute as each day passed, until it became a permanent and absolute state of being. Inevitably as I began to miss more and more lectures and I fell behind in my studies, everything compounded on top of me and I was again rapidly losing my ability to cope or even to comprehend what was happening to me.

Similar to when I had been at Kent, initially I still tried to function in the evenings, when the day was over and when I felt less guilty and anxious about the fact that I was not at lectures or studying. I could still just about relate to others at these times. I took some small comfort (or was it transference) in the fact that James was really hating his course in Quantitative Surveying; a subject that he had quickly come to realise he had absolutely no interest in. One evening in a moment of complete madness or group hysteria, we decided we would both leave polytechnic and start a new life in America. What we would do there was immaterial, maybe we would clean windows, but we would enjoy life away from the pressures of studying. At that point James was probably almost as bat-shit crazy as I was, but he managed to keep it together and gave me lots of support throughout the extended periods of desperation and anguish that were rushing towards me at full speed[4].

---

[4] At the end of James' first year, he transferred from Quantitative Surveying to a degree in English.

Down Down........

After only a few weeks of feeling relatively normal at Polytechnic I had plummeted to depths of depression I had never imagined existed, added to this my self-esteem had gone subterranean as I started to face the very real chance that I was about to drop out of Higher Education for the second time in under a year. I really thought I was losing my mind at that time. I couldn't think clearly and barely managed to cope beyond those tasks required for keeping myself alive. In this state one morning, I went out to find a cash point machine to get some money to go buy a train ticket to get me home to Frimley Green. As I tried to navigate the streets, I was sweating profusely, I felt as if I couldn't function on any level any longer, I couldn't focus on where I was going or what I was doing, and I could only see black all around me. I think I was then at my lowest ever mental state. The hot sweats and panic attacks got worse and worse over the next few days and I decided to pack my bags and head home once again. I was still desperately trying to hold onto something; I took with me some of my books and lecture notes in the hope that I could study back in Frimley Green. Who was I kidding? I could not decipher or follow anything I took with me, and I began to resign myself to a failed life. I was only trying to hold on to my sanity as I was determined not to end up in a mental institution or to kill myself as my mother had done. Once back at home I sat watching TV and crying, receiving comfort of sorts from my grandmother who really didn't grasp what I was going through. If I'd had different more aware guardians, or had there been two of them to discuss my plight (my grandfather for obvious reasons didn't count) maybe they would have contacted a doctor immediately and I could have received some much-needed professional intervention, but my grandmother just thought I was going through some kind of phase, she had after all witnessed my mother going through a lot of similar phases!

This time being back at home was worse than before; my friends were away studying, I had no-one I could turn to and I felt utterly and completely alone. There were sporadic visits from my Uncle Vernon, who had by then become a pharmaceutical sales rep with seemingly a lot of spare time on his hands (presumably this was an indicator of how busy he was at work), and I visited my Auntie Myra who after separating from Vernon, was living with her dog Heathcliff in a council flat in Aldershot. These visits did help a bit and I enjoyed the silent company of Myra and Heathcliff. There must have been some small crumb of self-preservation in me that was still intact, as this time I wasn't so stupid as to sever my links with the polytechnic completely and had instead signed myself off sick. I was back on the anti-depressants in the vain hope that they would bring me back from the precipice; they never did. I was just about holding onto some a thin slice of myself and was waiting for Keith and Tim to return from their studies so that I could at least spend time with friends over Christmas. That was my only thought and as far ahead as I could manage to see, I wasn't capable of thinking or planning any further than that.

...Deeper and down

I don't recall much of Christmas '82 although I know that I spent lots of time with Keith's parents, who I had come to think of as my surrogate family. I also saw a lot of Tim's family as well as Vernon, Myra, and my cousins, Chris and Julie. I would go and see anyone that had a kind word for me and a shoulder to cry on. Thank God these people were there for me in my time of need, I don't like to think about what could have happened if they hadn't been. In my depressed state I was only concerned with getting through each day, and every night I went to bed and hoped to not wake up the following day. Sleeping brought me no solace as I dreamed of the great times I had had as a child, only to be replaced each morning when I woke with the reality of the nightmare life I was now living.

Christmas was soon over and it was time for Keith and Tim to go back to their colleges. I was envious of the normal lives they were leading and maybe that's what panicked me into returning to poly' for the start of the next academic term. Believing that I had pretty much blown my degree course again, I thought that I could try and convince the relevant authorities to let me change to a Diploma course, I would do any subject they offered me. This was fantastical thinking on my part, no doubt influenced by my condition and the absence of any alternative, but I was simply unwilling to believe that I couldn't cope with a Maths Higher National Certificate, never mind an HND or a degree course in something. Of course, I had still not grasped that it wasn't the studying that was making me ill, it was my illness that made the studying impossible. I don't think it would have made any difference what subject or level of course I took at the time, my illness was not going to let me do it.

In desperation and spurred on by a minor uplift in my mood and energy levels during the Christmas period which had left me feeling marginally better emotionally, I thought that if I could somehow battle on and keep going, I might just be able to pull myself onto a higher plane than I was currently on and manage my way out of my depression. I had yet to appreciate the learning that I stated at the start of this book that having a bipolar condition is an illness, and in many cases, just like with a physical illness, without the appropriate interventions i.e. medication in my case, the condition will run its own course and to a large extent recovery timescales are outside of your control. Anyway, I had nowhere else to go and this was a last roll of the dice. Tim, being Tim, generously offered to drive me back to polytechnic and also to help me search for new digs, since I had by then withdrawn from residential accommodation provided by the poly'. I was aware that I had become increasingly reliant, dependant even, on others around me to help me deal with things that until relatively recently I would have taken in my stride. I hoped that maybe someday I would return to my old independent ways and be able to return this kindness but at that moment in time I was in need and I was simply grateful to have people around me who cared sufficiently to help.

On arriving at the polytechnic with Tim, we immediately went to see the Dean of the Faculty, a very pleasant lady who undoubtedly had more experience and understanding of my situation than I at first appreciated. Despite my imploring her to look at different solutions that might work better for me and my illness at that time, she held firm to the position that I must come back and start the new term on the course I was signed up to, and she stated that it was just not possible for me to switch courses. I don't remember any other offers of pastoral support being mentioned and it is a possibility that the Dean, seeing the hopelessness of my plight, was more interested in limping me through to the next data census point that would enable the college to at least draw down their next tranche of government funding for my fees; although maybe that is me being overly cynical. Either way, this was absolutely not what I wanted to hear. I left the Dean's office feeling distraught as things were not going according to plan. Tim did his best to reassure me that this was a positive thing since I was still on my course and although I was desperate for any reassurance I could get, I didn't feel comforted or reassured. The Dean had given us a few addresses provided by the student union of possible places for me to live; the first of which was a multi-story block of flats in Woolwich.

It was quite late in the afternoon when we got to the flat but I was exhausted and desperate for somewhere to stay that night as well as to secure some semi-permanent digs for the new term. A very friendly middle-aged woman opened the door, let us in, and showed us around. I managed to make some small talk and was able to hold myself together enough to give the impression that I was an honest enough guy who would make a reliable tenant. It was a small flat with two bedrooms, an open plan kitchen/lounge, and its major redeeming feature was a fantastic view looking down into the city of London. Incredibly, the woman agreed to let us stay the night and to sort out the finances for payment of the rent the next day. She was clearly delighted, believing she had found a model tenant, and outwardly we both appeared very satisfied with the arrangement. On the inside though I was far from happy and fast approaching a total meltdown at the thought of living in this flat alone. That night Tim slept on the floor and I had the bed, and the next morning, after the landlady had left for work leaving us to let ourselves out, I scribbled her a note; thanking her profusely, but apologising and explaining that I had decided for personal reasons i.e. I had just gone mad, that I was not going to return to polytechnic, and wouldn't need the room after all. And there and then my Higher Education ambitions came to an abrupt end!

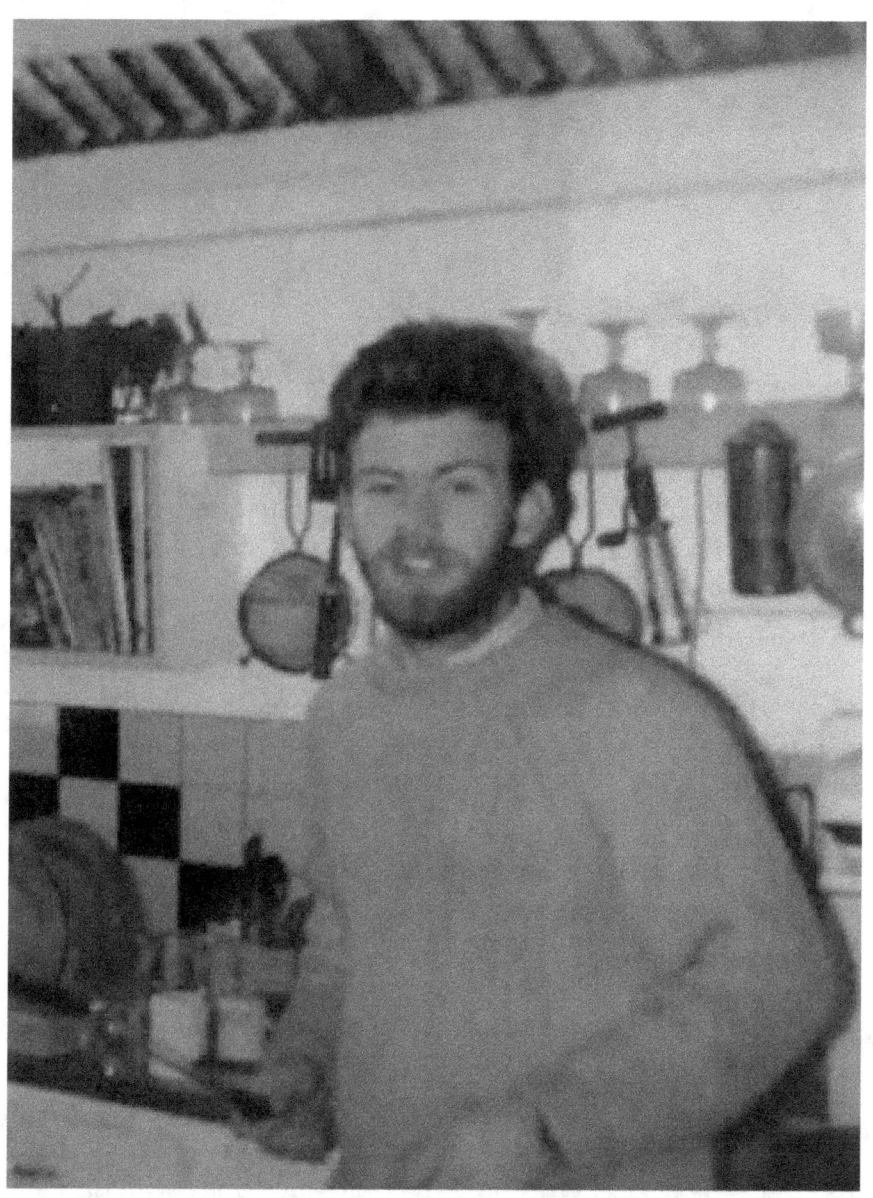

Tim in his kitchen in Bangor, I can never repay him for the kindness and support he gave me when I left Thames Poly.

Chapter 8 - From pillar to post

Bangor, January 1983

My terror at the thought of being left alone in London, extended to the prospect of returning to the grim reality and isolation of Frimley Green. Tim, sensing this, asked me if I would like to stay with him for a while when he went back to Bangor University in a few days' time. Without a moment's hesitation I said yes and so a couple of days later I found myself in Tim's digs in a decidedly cold North Wales; although I may have been mentally and emotionally dead, my physical senses assured me that my corporeal body was bloody freezing. Tim, having always been a bit maverick and independent minded, had moved out of his comfortable shared accommodation in the city of Bangor and into a small bungalow on his own on the beautiful nearby island of Anglesey. The main attraction for the move I assumed must have been a low rent as it certainly wasn't for the amenities. The house was allegedly kept warm by electric storage heaters, which perversely accumulated heat at night when the electricity was cheaper, BUT when you were in most need of being kept warm, they then belted out heat during the day, which was when Tim and I were frequently out. Tim looked after me very well while I stayed with him, as well as attending to his own studies (I could have done with his calm role model and companionship when I had been at Kent or Thames).

I got to see quite a bit of Bangor as I accompanied Tim to University when he attended his lectures which were spread across different sites across the town. Tim showed me some of the beautiful sights of Anglesey, Snowdonia, and North Wales, but I was not in the right frame of mind to appreciate them; It would have been a much more enjoyable experience for me, had I not been clinically depressed, psychotic, and on the brink of a nervous breakdown. When walking over the magnificent and historic Menai Bridge all I thought was "if I jumped off this, I could kill myself and all my troubles would be over". But there was no real likelihood of this as I was too cowardly and my self-preservation instinct still pulled me through each day. I cannot thank Tim enough for his thoughtfulness and kindness and for a while I became like his second shadow not wanting to leave his side. We went to the zoo and the cinema, I remember we saw Rambo, First Blood with Sly Stallone, and one evening we went to a disco, where in spite of everything I managed to have a couple of dances and even a kiss with a girl. That night, somewhere deep inside me, the memory of this first intimate experience I had had with a girl for several years made me think that if only I could get well again life could be okay and normal. That was wishful thinking as I think normality, a largely foreign concept to me at the best of times, was a long way off and I would have to endure a lot of pain and trauma first before I got there - but I had to have hope.

Hannover

After three weeks in Bangor, Tim drove me back home to Frimley Green and to my grandparents. My grandmother, probably being less than thrilled at the prospect of having a morose me hanging around, in addition to a morose grandfather, immediately suggested that I might benefit from a complete change by visiting my Aunt Elga, my Uncle Stennie, and my cousins, Mario and Daniel, in Hannover, Germany. Still feeling far from well enough to contemplate reassembling my life and also keen to extend my break from my grandmother's shouting and screaming, I agreed to go.

I don't know how I managed to cope with the journey to Hannover as I was a bag of nerves when I set off from Frimley Green. The journey required me to catch a train to London Waterloo, navigate the confusing and hectic London Underground to get to Liverpool Street, and then take another train to Harwich where I would get the ferry to the Hook of Holland and from there yet another train to Hannover. What in other circumstances would have felt like an exhilarating adventure, left me almost rigid with fear and anxiety. Throughout the journey I blocked out the outside world by keeping my headphones locked to my head and listening to music on my Sony Walkman. This way I maintained a closed reality that consisted almost exclusively of my own bleak thoughts and feelings. As a consequence, whenever I think back to that nightmare journey, my memories are always accompanied by a soundtrack of David Bowie, Eurythmics, Yazoo, Brian Eno, Jeff Wayne, Lou Reed, and other rock and roll legends; as I said it was a long journey.

I had never before met my Uncle Stennie and his family as they had always lived in Germany. Stennie met me at the train station and drove me to his home. On arriving at Stennie's I found that enough of my confidence had returned for me to string a few introductory sentences together. My cousins, Mario and Daniel, both spoke quite good English, but fortunately for me, not so good that they were able to pick up that I was struggling to speak my own language coherently. Both boys were close to my own age and both had jobs or apprenticeships and lived what seemed to me to be full and active social lives. During my stay, I met several of their friends when we went to bars and discos, and although I didn't understand a lot of what was being said, I found their joking and banter enjoyable and recuperative (despite my preconceptions about the German sense of humour). Stennie and Elga were wonderful hosts and did everything they could to make me feel at home and amongst a loving family whilst I was there. During my stay, something within me changed, or at least began to change. Somehow being in this foreign environment, being cared for by loved ones, who importantly were my kin, together with the total lack of responsibility, little by little helped ease my depression and anxiety, so much so that by the end of my three week stay in Germany I returned home to the UK, in a better frame of mind than I had been for the last six months.

Shaun, Motorcycle City and the road back

Having returned to Frimley Green from Germany, I found myself once again living the familiar stultifying daily routines that I had come to know so well, an existence that sucked any remaining spirit I had left out from within me and left me feeling like a husk. Together with my grandmother, grandfather and Peter we would all sit for hours on end, day after day, hunched around the fire, staring into space in virtual silence lost in our own thoughts and torments. At least they were reliving life time's full of rich memories as they moved towards the end of their lives, whereas I still felt as if mine had yet to begin. Any salvation for me was definitely not going to come from this direction. Thankfully Shaun wasn't around much any longer as he had a pregnant girlfriend and he spent a lot of time with her. This was okay with me as I didn't really have the energy for Shaun and despite our much-improved relationship, I was still wary of how changeable he could be, and I didn't think my fragile ego could stand a further onslaught from him at that time. Shaun was still working at Motorcycle City and he had let them know that I was back in circulation; they had reported back that they could use me if I was interested. Initially this prospect troubled me immensely, but I forced myself to acknowledge that if I was to have any hope of rebuilding my life, I had to start by getting the hell out the house during the day. From somewhere I found enough energy and motivation to take them up on this offer and returned with my tail firmly between my legs to Motorcycle City. Many of my old colleagues were still there and they treated me kindly and respectfully, as evidenced by their behaviour towards me, which was much the same as it had been before I left. Gradually over time, now that I was back in the Motorcycle City gang, doing something and meeting people again, my mental state improved sufficiently for me to reduce and eventually come off my anti-depressants, and commence a more natural recovery. Every day I felt a bit better; one day at a time I gradually recovered my faculties.

After a couple of months at Motorcycle City I was offered the chance to come off payment by piece rate and instead to move onto a permanent full-time contract, which I accepted with open arms. As a full-time bike builder earning a regular salary instead of being paid per bike, I became more relaxed at work and wasn't subject to the pressure of having my earnings related directly to my output. I was trying not to think too much about the future and for the time being just to live in the moment. I had money, not much, but I didn't have many outgoings; oh, and Shaun had moved out to live with his girlfriend. With life having returned to some kind of semi-normality and manageable patterns, the next few months remained relatively calm and I found myself back in the same situation pretty much where I had been 12 months previously, although I now had another strike against my name.

Summer of '83, Motorcycle City and some get rich quick wheeling and dealing.

By about May 1983, I had started socialising outside of work with my colleagues from Motorcycle City. On my trips to the workshop for parts or tools, I would chat with a young girl called Anita, who to my delight told me she had recently split up from her long-term boyfriend. Always one to take whatever advantage I could from someone else's misfortune, I asked her out there and then; and amazingly she agreed. It was to be my first proper date for years. The date was largely unmemorable, although I do recall that things got a little frisky in the front of my car; we stayed friendly after this date, but we never went out together again. Although Anita was only a little older than me, she was certainly more experienced and I guess I didn't measure up. Never mind at least I was back in the game and I was optimistic that there would be more opportunities with the opposite sex in the future.

Now that the financial situation regarding my grandparents' house had been stabilised and I was no longer having to make repayments on the loan my uncle had taken out, I had much more disposable income; so, I bought myself a second-hand car. Again, not a very good one, nor a very practical one; it was a six-cylinder Triumph 2000TC, which did about 20mpg if I was lucky. The previous owner had used it as a taxi which should have made me suspicious of the amazingly low mileage on the clock; but I didn't care. It was big, it was brash, it was fun to drive, and it looked the business. I think I justified it to myself at the time since I only intended to keep it for a short while, sell it for a profit, and then buy a more boring practical car. A colleague at work had recently done something similar with a Pontiac Firebird and someone else with a Corvette, and the end results were transformational and turned a significant profit.

The work at Motorcycle City was beginning to become routine and I found that my motivation and enthusiasm was waning and somewhat to my surprise I had begun having thoughts of moving on. What to? I had no idea: I had certainly burned all my bridges as far as Higher Education was concerned. But my confidence was in the ascendency once more, probably running ahead of me, as I was convinced that something would come along (see Bipolar symptoms book 101). I was full of energy running six miles three or four times a week, on top of which I was cycling about 50 miles a week, to and from work. To break up the monotony at work, I took on a bet with several colleagues that I could eat 50 raw eggs (a challenge inspired through having recently watched Paul Newman in the film Cool Hand Luke). I was feeling fit and strong and more than equal to the task as I had already tested myself with an earlier trial run of 25 eggs. Also, I had found a place where I could buy pullet eggs, which were much smaller than chicken eggs. But alas, pride comes before a fall and I think I must have become overconfident, as the night before the day of the challenge I had been to the pub and drank a number of pints. I blame the bloating effect of the beer from the night before as the reason why I threw up after only thirty-seven eggs. It was not a pretty sight. Not only did I lose the bet but I felt absolutely terrible for the rest of the day. I lost about £100 in total (over a week's wages); it would have been more had it not been for the fact that I had taken some side bets with lower odds, with punters who thought that I wouldn't make it past 25 eggs (my first dabbling in the investment strategy of hedging).

My next fantastical scheme was buying an old pick-up truck; following my fool proof plan to buy it cheap, do it up, and sell it on for a profit. Hey if I could put the wheels and handlebars on a motorbike, in my mind (at that time) I could do anything.

The truck was in a terrible condition, which was reflected in the asking price. My fanciful restoration projects had earned me something of a reputation as an easy mark amongst my colleagues at Motorcycle City; if you had a pile of shit to get rid of, offload it on Marcus, he'll even pay you for it). Of course, this latest plan never got off the ground either, and having bought the truck I only got as far as giving it a dodgy respray and then when it failed its MOT, because surprise surprise, most of its body panels were as thin as cardboard, and may even have been made out of cardboard, I lost interest. Had anyone been monitoring my behaviour at this time and perhaps plotting it on a chart, it is a fair bet that it would suggest that I was on an upward trajectory in my bipolar mood swings at this time. I had thrown myself into a number of entrepreneurial schemes starting with the sale of my beloved Yamaha SR500 and ending with the disposal of a heap of shit, non-road worthy pickup truck. But I was not disillusioned, Elon Musk a fellow bipolar sufferer, experienced a number of business setbacks before he went on to become one of the richest men in the world. It did seem however that some aspects of my bipolar condition i.e. the increased appetite for risk, ill-considered fantastical ideas; were influencing my judgement and decision making, as I sought to turn a profit from my various get rich quick schemes, but which had so far only succeeded in making a loss.

By the end of June that year, I became unexpectedly unemployed when I was given the sack from Motorcycle City for being absent from work without permission. To cut a long story short I had been invited to go and stay with Tim at his parents who were now living in Fareham in Hampshire. Visiting Tim at his parents was one of my favourite things in the world; I loved to see Tim and his family, I helped out around the house by doing DIY projects with Tim's dad, and best of all, Tim and I would go swimming in the sea at Hayling Island and then round off the day with a couple of pints at a local pub. It was as close to paradise as anything I had ever known. On the Thursday before the day I planned to drive to Fareham, I informed Neil my foreman that I was going to take the Friday off (okay, I was only giving him one day's notice, and maybe I should have asked his permission rather than simply advising him of my intentions). Not surprisingly, Neil said no. But I wasn't going to let a little thing like that stop me, so I went anyway. When I turned up for work again on the Monday morning, I was told I no longer had a job. Although this wasn't the way I would have chosen to end things, I wasn't overly worried; by then the shine had gone off the job for me, I was growing bored with the work and as I regained my confidence and self-esteem, I believed that I was destined for greater things, so I was pretty sanguine about getting sacked. For the record, the weekend at Tim's was everything I hoped it would be and I remember it to this day. Losing my job didn't faze me in the least because I was once again high on life, the summer was coming, and I thought that as long as I put my mind to it, the next job, which would be far more suited to my skills and knowledge, was waiting just around the corner for me.

Chapter 9 - The power of love

The summer of 1983 was notable again for its consistent warm weather and I remember July and August as being swelteringly hot. In August, Tim came back from the South Coast for a visit and together with Keith we visited some of our old haunts. I went back with Tim to Fareham as there couldn't be a better time to be by the coast than during the summer months. Tim and I went to a party near Woking of some mutual school friends from St John the Baptist, Irish twins Eamonn and Phil Farrelly. Tim drove and it was great to remake old acquaintances and catch up on what was happening in their lives, although naturally I was a little reticent about talking about my years since leaving St Johns. After a little while I began talking to the cutest and most gorgeous girl that I can remember. She had been to St Tar's and to St John's but had been in the year below me, and so I had never really spoken with her previously. My how she had changed! This was Jackie Washington, who was to become my first serious girlfriend. I learned that after her A-levels, Jackie had deferred her university place for a year; choosing instead to get some work experience behind her, which she was currently doing by working as a PA at an Estate Agents in Camberley. At the end of the summer Jackie was going to Leeds University to study English. We chatted and danced with each other all night and as the drink flowed and our conversation got more intimate, Jackie gave my ego a great boost by saying that she, and several of her friends, had always fancied me at school, but they had viewed me as being a bit aloof and superior at that time. I had not had too much time for romance towards the end of my time at SJB, since as you already know these were my table-tennis years when girls were just a distraction. One negative consequence of which was that I had never really learned how to talk to or behave in front of girls at the time, so maybe this is what Jackie had mistaken for aloofness on my part. We continued to dance close together for the rest of the evening and our intimacy progressed to include kissing and cuddling. At the end of the party to my delight, we exchanged contact details and agreed to meet again soon.

Love is the drug

Although by most benchmarks I was still in a far from settled state i.e., I was still living with my grandparents, I was unemployed, and there was nothing in the pipeline; one big thing in my favour was my buoyant mental state. Whereas before living with my grandparents added to my depression, I now saw their arguments as banter and felt able to join in; trying to take some of the sting out of my grandmother's criticisms of my grandad and Uncle Peter. I took an interest in Uncle Vernon's visits (which had become quite frequent since things were not going well for him professionally or domestically), and also in the steady stream of strangers coming to see my grandmother to have their cards read and their fortunes told. The good weather helped buoy my spirits up and I kept myself busy with odd jobs around the house; added to this of course I was now in love and in my first proper relationship, with Jackie Washington. I was like a child at the time I simply couldn't hear her name spoken out loud enough times. I felt consistently happy for the longest time since before my mother died. Once again, I was living in and for the moment, and I had put all thoughts or long-term planning on the back burner. If things stayed as they were at that point forever, that would be okay by me.

I quickly learned that Jackie was very ambitious and determined to prove that it wasn't only the men in her family that could be successful: Jackie's brother, Mick, owned a building company and was involved in some prestigious developments in London; I think secretly Jackie wanted to prove herself as capable, if not more so, than Mick. At the end of the summer Jackie was to head off to Leeds University to study English, and shortly before she left we went on holiday together to the South of France. This was a sublime holiday and we just bathed in the sun and the sea together, got to know each other a lot better, and just chilled out without a care in the world. I wished it would never end, although Jackie was really looking forwards to going to uni' in September.

Love was my drug and in the state of mind I was in, I thought it inconceivable that I could ever relapse into a depressive state again. If things slipped a bit, Jackie and I could turn the love dial up a notch or two and all would be well. But sadly, once again I was about to be reminded that this was not how being bipolar works, my illness would decide when it came again, and it wasn't about to let a little thing like my love life or my apparent happiness stand in its way.

Slow train crash coming, back to reality

Before Jackie went away to university, she had asked her brother Mick if he could use me at all in the family building business, and Mick had generously agreed to take me on as a labourer. I am not sure that this was what I had in mind when I left Motorcycle City, when I imagined that I would move onto something more suited to my skill set; however, nothing else had come my way and with Jackie's departure imminent, my prospects were beginning to look and feel a bit bleak, so I gratefully accepted Mick's kind offer. Things must have been on the move again in my mental state because far from the "I can do anything" confidence that I had felt at the start of the summer, I harboured secret concerns that the work with Mick would prove too much for me. But I took the job anyway as I needed the money as well as something to do, and psychologically I felt that I would remain closer to Jackie through my daily involvement with her family. Mick's gang of workers were a motley crew consisting of his brothers, brother in-law, and close friends. I got on particularly well with Steve, who was married to Jackie's sister, Sue. Steve was the carpenter of the gang, and like many carpenters who have to wait for the different trades to finish their work before they can move in, he had made himself competent in several other aspects of building so as to be kept busy, and his second specialist skills was plastering.

The gang of blokes working for Mick were paid extremely well in relation to the market rates, and I understood this to be because of the high expectations placed on them by Mick to work efficiently, effectively, and to a very high quality on the more prestigious jobs that Mick secured. They worked predominantly on house renovations in up and coming areas of London, which were subject to gentrification during the 1980's. The job they were working on when I started was a renovation job on a large Victorian House in Notting Hill Gate. As well as the more standard renovation work, this job involved completely gutting the place prior to renovation and then excavation for an indoor swimming pool in the extension. This luxury conversion job looked like it would keep Mick and his merry band of men busy for at least 12 months.

Like labourers all over the country, I was picked up each morning at daybreak from outside my house, half asleep I would tumble into the van and return home again about 12 hours later, filthy and exhausted. Mick's pride and joy was his big blue pick-up truck, which could take all seven of us. Three lucky guys got to ride comfortably up front in the cab, whilst the rest of us rattled around in third class in the back without the luxury even of a roof or seats. The long journey to and from London added over three hours to our working day, and after a knackering eight hours of labouring I would often fall into an uncomfortable sleep in the truck on the way home. As the youngest, newest and certainly least skilled team member, most of the time I acted as a labourer and gofer for Steve. By then I could sense that my depression was on its way back again, but I tried my best to engage with Steve's attempts at conversation as he was such a friendly and happy go lucky guy. For the first couple of months, I managed to hide how I was feeling, although I had begun pulling back from the group banter that was such an important part of being in the team. Instead of joining in with the chat during tea breaks or the lunch hour, I would keep myself to myself making an excuse of going for a walk or nipping off to buy a sandwich. I had begun again to feel incapable of holding my own socially and the group conversations became the most challenging and difficult parts of the day for me. Once more the familiar feelings of numbness, inability to think clearly, and the terrifying thoughts of being on a precipice with my life falling apart were my constant daily companions. As I wandered aimlessly through the streets of Notting Hill, looking without seeing into the windows of the shops, I knew instinctively how the illness would soon drain me absolutely of energy and render me incapable of doing even the simplest of things. I tried to tell myself that whilst the labouring job was physically demanding, it wasn't intellectually challenging, most of it was very repetitive in nature and I just had to find the energy and the willpower to carry on. My low mood would pass... it must pass, and then I would feel better again. I had to keep going; I needed the job, I needed the money, and it was Jackie's brother I was working for. I couldn't show my weakness to her family and I couldn't let Jackie down after the faith she had shown in me. Somehow, although each day was sheer torture, I managed to make it through to Christmas when Jackie returned from Leeds. Ironically Mick had told Jackie that he thought I showed great potential and could easily master a trade if I put my mind to. I was touched by Mick's comments, but little did Mick know that I was not even master of my own mind, which chose to do what it wanted, when it wanted.

Interview with the BBC

It was Christmas 1983 and Jackie was back from university. I was holding things together as well as I could, but I was still not sharing how I was really feeling as I didn't want Jackie to worry and I still hoped that if I could just bluff it for long enough, I would start coming out of my depression and she would be none the wiser. At the time, knowing that I wanted to pursue a career that I thought more befitting my intellectual skills, Jackie encouraged me to apply for a job she had seen advertised for a BBC trainee cameraman. Jackie felt that on paper I was a reasonably good fit for this position, and so long as I doctored my past a little, edited out my failures at university and polytechnic, avoided any reference to my mental health, and lied about my interest in cinematography (which in reality had ended at the age of 16 when I took my O-level in photography), I was just what they were looking for. In fact, as long as I said nothing about anything I had done since leaving school aged 18, I was in with a chance. I duly applied, adhering to this minimalist principle (most of my future job applications were based on a similar policy of being both highly creative and yet economic with the truth when it came to my past) and when I had finished, I didn't recognise myself amongst the morsels of truth remaining in my application. It came as a great surprise to me when a few weeks later, I received a letter offering me a first interview. My technical knowledge from my O-level photography served me sufficiently well and I managed to answer all the questions they asked on exposure settings, focal lengths, lighting etc; and so, the farce continued when I was invited back for a second interview. The second interview proved to be the point where they really sorted the wheat from the chaff and it quickly became apparent to the interviewers that the knowledge I had demonstrated in my first interview wasn't just the tip of the iceberg, it was the iceberg itself. My superficial knowledge was excruciatingly exposed, as was the fact that I was out of my depth, totally inexperienced, and nowhere near responsible enough for the role. Still, on the plus side, I think that I managed to hide from them the fact that I was mentally ill.

Breaking point and self-admission to psychiatric ward of Frimley Park Hospital – February 1984

After the Christmas break, Jackie returned to Leeds and I went back to work, but I just couldn't keep up the pretence that I was coping any longer and one afternoon when Mick was leaving the site early, I went up to him and told him that I wasn't feeling well, and that I needed to go home. With just Mick and I in the truck on the way back to Frimley Green, I broke down. Not for the first time in my life I found myself sobbing uncontrollably, and in between the tears and the snot, I let it all out to Mick, opening up about all my problems and saying that that I simply could no longer cope with the job. Mick was extremely sympathetic and supportive and as I got out of the truck he told me to take as much time as I needed to get better. Up until that point, the Washington family with the exception of Jackie were unaware of my illness and past and I had not even told Jackie that I feared I was spiralling downwards again. She had accepted my spin about how I had grown out of my illness and was now a well-balanced, if a little carefree, normal young man. After speaking with Mick, I used the pay-phone in the relative privacy of the working man's club where my grandfather worked, to call Jackie and tell her everything. It was a great relief to finally be honest with her. Jackie agreed that I should go to the doctor's urgently and seek some kind of professional help and longer term treatment. It was now apparent that my cycles of depression were independent of my environment, which suggested that there might be something clinically wrong with me. This was something of a turning point for me really, and I am surprised that it had taken me so long to reach that place of self-realisation and to finally acknowledge that I might not be able to beat this thing on my own.

Once again, my prospects were looking pretty bleak, but perhaps for the first time, with Jackie's words in my head, I was being proactive about my illness and the next day I made an appointment to see my GP. I told him that I had come to the end of the line; although it felt dramatic saying it out loud, I remember thinking, in for a penny in for a pound, and I went on to say that the way things were I couldn't face another day[5]. Dr Bartlett (my friend Tom's father) recommended that I admit myself voluntarily to the psychiatric ward at Frimley Park hospital, to undergo a week's observation in order to get a fuller assessment of my condition. I found some comfort in this suggestion as it was encouraging to have my situation acknowledged by a doctor and also, I relished the potential prospect of finding out what was wrong with me, as a first step

---

[5] I should clarify that although several times during the repeated depressions in my illness, I felt as if couldn't go on and would rather be dead, I never felt that I would take my own life - this is a significant distinction, and I don't believe I was ever a suicidal risk.

towards putting things right. Finally, I wouldn't have to hide myself away in my small room at my grandparents, alone with my blackness, waiting and hoping for some small sign that my condition was improving. I would be supported by professionals, who would be of more help to me than the well-intentioned but helpless words of comfort from my grandmother. I had begun to feel increasingly alone and frightened about my future, since my illness had seemed to be getting worse; the lows were becoming lower, the highs were becoming higher, and the swings seemed to be increasing in frequency. Now I would have the support of others, I didn't have to go through it on my own anymore; surely that at least was positive news.

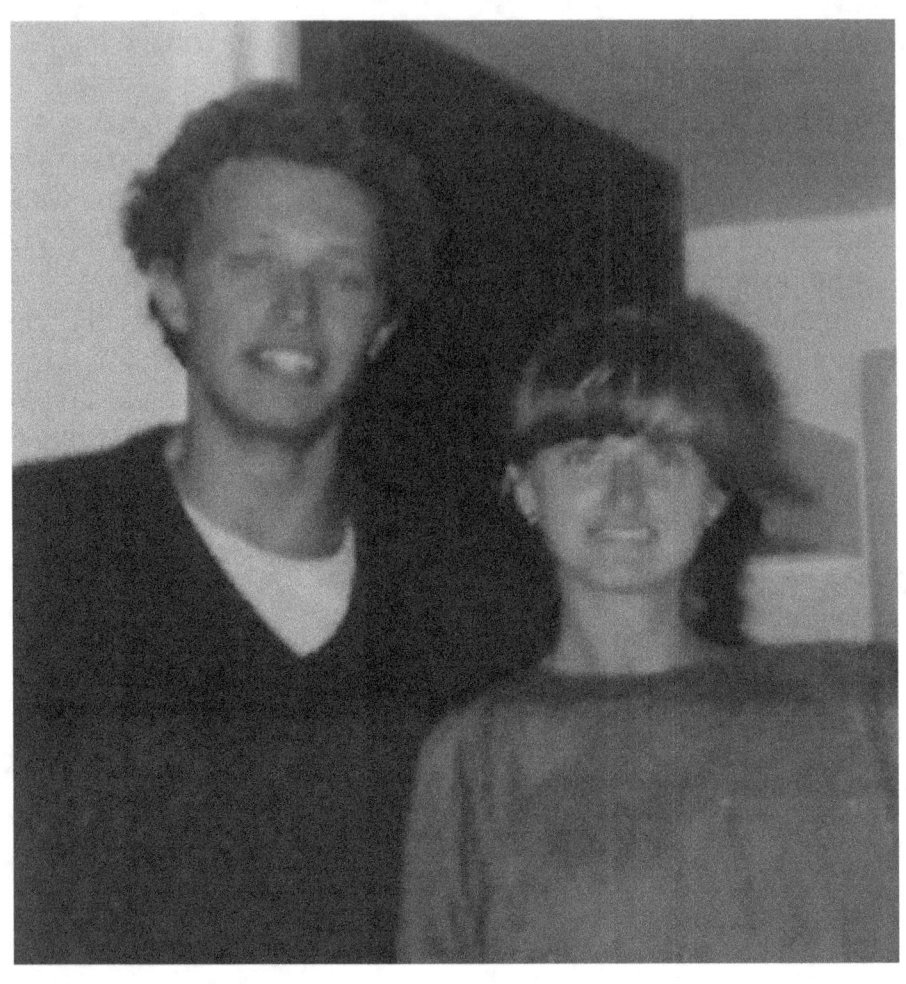

Jackie and myself looking very young.

Chapter 10 - Self admission to a psychiatric ward

Frimley Park Hospital is a large general hospital in Frimley in Surrey. It opened in 1974 and included in its services a psychiatric ward. This was where I found myself one afternoon back in February 1984; feeling apprehensive, scared, and not having a clue about what was about to happen next. My referral had been arranged via Dr Bartlett, and when I arrived at the hospital, I was met by a nurse who took me to the psychiatric ward. I said an emotional goodbye to my grandmother who appeared very eager to get back into the taxi and return home. For a short while I waited in a chair in the ward hallway until I was taken to the canteen and given a specially selected meal; I was famished and quickly finished the lot. After the meal I was taken to a small side room and told a doctor would be along to see me shortly. The doctor arrived about five minutes later in a white coat and asked me to sit on a bed; he proceeded to ask me a few questions, including questions about my personal life. It seemed very odd to me when his questions included; "Who is the Queen of England?" followed by "What year is it?" and then, "What month is it?". I presume that from the outset he wanted to establish just how in touch with reality I was. This questioning struck me as silly and I began laughing crazily, way out of proportion to the oddness of the situation; so much so that when I got control of myself again, I looked at the doctor and asked him what had been put in my food to make me feel so weird and behave this way? The doctor looked at me without any hint of humour in his expression and replied that they had not put anything in my food. I reflected on his answer and thought worriedly to myself that I may know who the Queen of England was, but I am seriously beginning to doubt my grasp on reality.

Throughout the rest of the assessment, I emphasised how much I wanted to get well again. I tried to explain that it was the extreme mood swings that I couldn't cope with. I told the psychiatrist that my childhood had been a happy one, one in which I used to wake up each morning looking forward to the day ahead. Although I didn't remember being too upset after my mother's death, I recalled that my feelings had begun to change around that time, but I had kept up a pretence and maintained a full attendance at school throughout. I had been told that the school had reported back to my grandmother that somewhat to their surprise I hadn't shown any obvious signs of upset or distress in the months after my mother's death. I went on unloading to the psychiatrist that what no-one had known at the time, because I hadn't told anyone, was that after my mother's death I had felt more closed off and unsure of myself. Getting up each morning had become harder and I had only managed to force myself to keep going to school because I didn't want to become another victim of my mother's death. I recounted to him that I had deliberately backed off from involvement with my mother in the years leading up to her death as subconsciously I recognised a need to create some distance between myself and the emotional roller-coaster experience that her life had become. As I told my story I was amazed that the doctor was very familiar with my mother's history and even seemed to have a full file on her, which he referred to as we spoke. What's more to my shock and horror, he seemed to be making direct links between her behaviour and my problems. This was scary stuff since I had always thought of my mother's issues as being far more severe and extreme than mine, after all she had made several suicide attempts and eventually succeeded in hanging herself. With these confusing thoughts still racing around my mind I was taken to a bed on the ward, the curtains drawn around me for privacy, and I was medicated to ensure that I would relax and rest; just like Randle McMurphy in One flew over the Cuckoo's Nest I thought to myself.

The final decision to admit myself to the hospital had been made about a week before during a consultation with my GP. What I had understood from that meeting was that staying in hospital for a week's observation would help the specialists to properly assess and diagnose my condition towards the goal of prescribing me with the appropriate medication and treatment to help make me better. After a week of this I would then be sent on my way, to live long and prosper; or so I thought! Perhaps Dr Bartlett had been a bit more circumspect in his explanation of what was likely to happen, I vaguely recalled him mentioning something about new treatments that might be suitable for me, which to my young ears was even more reason to hold out hope. During the first few days at hospital, I did not see another psychiatrist or psychologist, instead under the guidance of the nurses and the ebb and flow of the day's patterns, I adjusted into the routines and ways of life on the ward. Morning meds, followed by breakfast, followed by sitting about talking to a few other patients, followed by lunch, a sleep, a visitor (if I was lucky), tea, more meds and bed. I think at first the staff were experimenting with my drugs to see which worked best and were most suited to me. I don't recall what they were called, but the ones I started on gave me an incredibly dry mouth and made me so tired and exhausted that I could not think at all. I quickly complained about this and although my medication was changed, I was still kept waiting to see a psychiatrist.

By the end of my second week (hadn't Dr Bartlett said I would only be there for one week?) I had only seen a psychiatrist once in a 10-minute face-to-face consultation. He told me that it was possible that my mood instability may have been sparked by an event in my childhood, which could have caused an upset to my brain chemistry, which might have resulted in me becoming bipolar. In amongst all his tentativeness and speculation and qualifying words did I just hear some kind of a diagnosis of my illness; did he say bipolar? I immediately thought of my mother, and what I had always perceived as being her much more severe condition, and from these thoughts I drew my own conclusions on the spot. Namely, that I had inherited my mother's bipolar illness, I would have it forever, my life was over, I was fucked! The Doctor went on to say that based on this new hypothesis they were going to try a different approach to my medication and put me on lithium carbonate. Once again, my brain went racing.... I remembered lithium from my chemistry lessons at school, it's an alkali metal, number three in the periodic table, reacts violently with water, and is used in the production of batteries. How's that going to help me? After this bombshell had been dropped, I don't remember much more of what the doctor said and shortly afterwards he left me alone in the room with a thousand and one unanswered questions. Thankfully the nurses gave me a lot more information and reassurance on my proposed treatment, enlightening me on how the lithium worked, what my dosage meant, the importance of monitoring the amount of lithium in the blood stream to ensure it remained effective, and crucially also to avoid potentially damaging side effects to any of my organs.

Lithium has been used since the late 1800's to treat people with mania and it has become almost the drug of choice for the long-term treatment of people with bipolar. Lithium somehow acts as a mood stabiliser by interacting with the brain's neurotransmitters and neuron receptors. By and large

> *the effective pharmacological treatment of bipolar seems to suggest a combination approach in which a mood stabiliser (e.g. lithium) is combined with an anti-depressant (e.g. Prozac) to help with the extreme lows in the depressive state.*[6]

So, in my own personal take on things, it seemed to me that the net gain of these medications was to help prevent people with bipolar throwing themselves off bridges in attempts to kill themselves during severe depressions; or to prevent them throwing themselves off bridges thinking they can fly during extreme mania phases. If this explanation is insufficient for your needs, and why would it be, then go google, this narrative of my own personal experiences in no way serves as any kind of medical advice on the drug treatments used to manage the worst aspects of bipolar disorder.

My new world

During my first weeks in hospital, I got to know many of the other patients on the ward; including some who were there involuntarily, having been sectioned under the Mental Health Act. My days were mainly spent in the common room area where there was a TV, some books, and some board games, including my favourite - chess, although at first, I was in no fit state to meet the mental demands that any of these games demanded. I did make friends with three other younger patients, whose names I can't remember all these years later, but whose friendship was important to me at the time as they helped me make associations beyond myself. There was another young guy aged 18 who was in a pretty bad way and

---

[6] Antipsychotics are also sometimes prescribed in treating bipolar to help deal with some of the more extreme symptoms of mania and depressive states.

seemed to me to be getting worse not better. He had been an undergraduate at Cambridge University but had had a breakdown and was now in a psychotic state most of the time. Also, there was a young girl, who again I estimated to be in her late teens. She had a friendly personality and was bubbly and seemed full of life. I couldn't imagine what was wrong with her although I later learned that she was unable to sleep properly, and this really messed her up. The person I got closest to was a young girl, aged about seventeen or eighteen. She was suffering with the eating disorder bulimia. When she had first been admitted she had lost a huge amount of weight and had become dangerously ill as a consequence, but thankfully when I met her, she was in a more stable position. She and I would play cards and joke about in the evenings and I felt the stirrings of a physical attraction towards her. Fortunately for both of us, I was able to rationalise that she was a patient in a psychiatric ward and so was I, and this probably wasn't the best foundation for a stable relationship (oh and of course I already had a girlfriend who I loved deeply).

There were other patients who I also remember; a middle-aged lady who worked for the BBC who had had a nervous breakdown, and a builder in his early 40's whose relationship difficulties with his wife and daughter had led him to cut his wrists (having chatted with him I think this was more as a cry for help than because he sincerely wanted to end his life). There were lots of elderly patients whose minds appeared to have just burned out and they were suffering with dementia. I was no psychiatrist, but I couldn't imagine how these poor souls could become better regardless of treatment. And then there were those sad and disquieting individuals who appeared to have crossed over the divide into real insanity never to return, including a lady who had arrived, raving and in a straitjacket from Brookwood mental hospital (previously an asylum). Medication did enable her to eventually be calmed down but she always had a distant look in her eyes as if she remained firmly in a world separate to ours, constantly talking to people no one else could see (or at least I couldn't). Perhaps the saddest person I saw, who in other circumstances you could imagine should be the happiest person in the world, was a young woman who had totally withdrawn inside herself and was suffering from a severe case of post-natal depression. I hoped desperately, perhaps making connections with my own circumstances and my own mother, that with treatment she would become well enough to return home to love, care for, and nurture her young baby.

As the weeks in hospital slowly passed by, it was obvious that the seven-day observation period I had been led to expect seemed to be being extending indefinitely and none of the doctors or nurses were talking about me being discharged. I was by then feeling much better in myself, I couldn't tell if this was the effect of my medication or the normal pattern of shifting between the phases of my condition. Either way, to my surprise I found that I was in no hurry to leave; I kept telling myself just one more week, just one more week and then I'll be ready. I think I partly feared leaving the safety and routine of the hospital as this would mean returning to the scary outside world where I would have to become a real person again with all the responsibilities that involved; not least working out what on earth I was going to do with my life next.

The trip

Looking back now, after about four weeks on the ward, just like Jack Nicholson's character, McMurphy, in One Flew Over the Cuckoo's Nest, I was in danger of becoming too comfortable and institutionalised in the wards daily routines and my responsibility free existence in hospital. One day, several patients, including myself, volunteered to act as guinea pigs and travelled by minibus to the Brookwood mental hospital. Whilst there, we were to be questioned about our illnesses by trainee/junior mental health practitioners whose task, as part of their training, was to attempt a diagnosis i.e. put a name to our illness, and to suggest a treatment/medication regime. Included in the questions they asked us were, "do you have delusions of grandeur?", "do you ever hear voices in your head?", and "has any member of your family ever been admitted to a mental institution?". Although I answered no to the first two questions, I was able to confirm that indeed my mother had been admitted to this very same institution during her acute depressive states; and whilst here, amongst other treatments, she had been subjected to ECT[7]. By then, I had developed an unspoken fear that this controversial and barbaric form of treatment, which had been used on my mother, would be used on me. It had had no obvious positive lasting benefits with my mother, and any of you who have watched One Flew Over the Cuckoo's Nest will remember it's limited impact on Randle McMurphy. It took a full lobotomy to bring him under their institutional control and the direction of nurse Ratchett, God forbid that practice would find its way onto my treatment plan. That outing proved significant for me, the

---

[7] Electroconvulsive therapy (ECT) is a procedure, done under general anaesthesia, in which small electric currents are passed through the brain, intentionally triggering a brief seizure. ECT seems to cause changes in brain chemistry that can quickly reverse symptoms of certain mental health conditions. ECT often works when other treatments are unsuccessful and when the full course of treatment is completed, but it may not work for everyone. Much of the stigma attached to ECT is based on early treatments in which high doses of electricity were administered without anaesthesia, leading to memory loss, fractured bones and other serious side effects.

enjoyment of travelling though the leafy Surrey countryside combined with the sobering experience of being in the formidable Brookwood Hospital, reminded me that my stay at Frimley Park was temporary. It had by then fulfilled its objective of assessing and diagnosing my condition and establishing a long-term treatment regime, maybe it was time to start thinking about leaving, "put it in the basket chief".

The next step

Soon after my trip to Brookwood Hospital I received a visit from Uncle Vernon. He told me that he was going to be taking my cousin Chris, to an international fencing tournament in Cardiff. I knew that Keith would soon be finishing term at polytechnic in Pontypridd, South Wales, a short distance from Cardiff, so if I made a few calls I could get a lift with Vernon and Chris to Cardiff, and then go on by train to Ponty', as the locals affectionately call it. I looked on this as being the first real test of my ability to function again on my own in the outside world. When I arrived at Keith's digs, he introduced me to his house mates as they arrived back home at the end of the day. They were all very friendly and easy to get on with and Keith must have briefed them on my circumstances as no one asked any difficult or awkward questions. I felt quite comfortable in their company and I made a mental note as I held my own during all the joking around, that my communication and social skills had made a dramatic recovery. Amidst the copious amounts of beer that we consumed that weekend I got to know one of Keith's friends, Paul Nolan, pretty well. I was dossing down in a spare bed in Pauls' room and we discovered many common interests and experiences including music and touring holidays. Paul went on to become a close lifetime friend, who I have had many great times with in London and on holidays in the Czech Republic and the USA. To top it all off I managed to blag a lift back with Keith to the hospital as he was going home to revise for his exams. This relatively unremarkable trip to South Wales, was remarkable for me as it was the final push/proof that I was ready to leave hospital after what had turned out to be an eight-week stay.

Chapter 11 - Going home

Still more than a little apprehensive about what the future held for me, and with lots of jokes about how I hoped I wouldn't ever see the nurses and patients again (at least under those circumstances) I left hospital; my planned one-week stay had ended up as two months. Uncle Vernon picked me up and dropped me off at my grandparents' where I started on the next stage of my rehabilitation. During the next few months, my uncle, my cousins, and Myra did everything they possibly could in making me feel loved and wanted and to help me on my road to recovery. Significantly this included providing me with refuge when the histrionics and arguments between my grandparents were doing my head in and were too much to bear. For a while my routines and daily challenges were humdrum and more about consolidation than moving forwards e.g. waking up, eating breakfast, watching TV, reading the newspaper; but mundane suited me just fine, as I was looking to slowly but solidly reassemble myself as a functioning person first, then take stock and plan my next steps.

Of course, all this time I was also counting the days to when Jackie would return from university for the Summer. A lot had happened during the last twelve months since Jackie and I had met and started seeing each other; I couldn't help but reflect on her success and her families support and pride in her; whilst I felt that I had let mine down so badly, not just once but twice. How had I fallen so far in my standing, having gone from being top of the form to the bottom of the heap? These were depressing thoughts and best not dwelt on, so instead I tried to focus on what I did have, I had a beautiful girlfriend who I was very much in love with and who I would do my utmost to make happy and if at all possible, proud of me. At the time I don't think I realised how dependant my self-esteem had become tied to my relationship with Jackie; our relationship was one of the only things I had left which defined me in relation to something outside of just myself. Inadvertently though, through this sole focus, I was making myself vulnerable since everything that was good and positive in my life seemed to revolve around Jackie. I needed to start rebuilding the other aspects of my life, which felt doubly difficult as I perceived that I had burned my bridges with regards to any kind of decent career.

March '84 - A New Life

After returning home and gradually getting back into the swing of things I began to socialise with a few old school friends who were still living locally, and through one of these friends I managed to pick up some casual work with a company called Instant Muscle. At the time Instant Muscle were based in Farnham in Surrey and had been started by a local church minister, as an odd job firm that provided manual employment opportunities for young people. The tasks we carried out were mainly unskilled labouring, such as; garden clearing, painting fences, knocking down sheds, and filling skips, etc. The clue to the nature of the work was in the name really, we did the labour heavy type jobs that householders didn't want to do themselves and no self-respecting builder would lower themselves to do. But for me at the time, the work demanded quite a bit of physical effort i.e. the muscle, but it required very little thinking and presented very little mental stress for me. As far as I was concerned this was ideal since a) I was out of physical condition and b) I couldn't really think. Alongside this work, and with lots of encouragement from Jackie, I had started applying for permanent, albeit low level, administrative type jobs. Jackie had seen a vacancy for insurance clerks with Crown Life Insurance at their offices in Woking and once again with her support I applied. There was something about the job that appealed to me; not least that Woking itself was partly familiar to me as that was where I had spent five years of school at St John the Baptist. I was offered an interview and even though I told the interviewers that I knew nothing about insurance companies (an unusual and uncharacteristic piece of interview honesty on my part), they assured me that given my qualifications and maths skills I wouldn't have a problem learning all I needed to know. I was offered and accepted the job and the department I went to work in dealt with new applications for life insurance and my role was to process these applications and carry out initial underwriting checks. It was with a sense of shame that in several applications where the applicant had admitted to a mental illness or past treatment for mental ill health, I was obliged to turn them down automatically and decline them cover. The irony of this was not lost on me since it was only really as a result of finally acknowledging publicly and seeking professional help for my own mental ill health that I had been given the chance at rebuilding my own life and to become a functioning member of society again. Yet any mention by one of these applicants that they had done likewise was likely to be met with an automatic NO! Such is (or was) the stigma attached to mental ill health. I was always extremely cautious in any formal applications for anything, in particular job applications, about what I said about my mental health past.

I started in this relatively low-level responsibility role and things went okay, although whether as a result of my illness or my medication, I found that I had great trouble retaining information. I was constantly being admonished for forgetting important information and at the end of six months my probationary period was extended for a further six months as clearly the jury was still out on my longer-term suitability. I am grateful to Trevor and Barry, my managers, for sticking with me, as they would've been well within their rights to fire me. However as time went on, although I would still get confused and had problems focussing, gradually, perhaps as my medication became more balanced in my system, I started functioning more consistently and at a higher level. Initially I had been fearful of answering the telephone and speaking to agents about their queries regarding their client's applications, but little by little, I learned from listening in to how my colleagues dealt with these calls and I assimilated the language and jargon of the industry. I was still having problems remembering things particularly when on the phone though, and I was often too embarrassed to ask the caller to repeat information they had just given me; eventually for this reason it was suggested to me that I avoided answering the phone wherever possible. But with the passing of time, I sensed that I was adjusting better to the medication and I was affected by lack of concentration and confusion far less frequently. Most importantly, in a business that thrives on confidence, I was acquiring and retaining more knowledge, and this led to me feeling more confident in what I was doing and saying to others. Success breeds success as they say, and as my confidence steadily grew my work performance improved and I felt proud of the progress I had made, albeit in what was a fairly routine and basic job.

Now that I was feeling more secure in my job, I felt able to replace my rusty, red ford escort estate with a much newer ex company car - another ford escort estate (I could only cope with so much change). Things were generally improving for me and once more Jackie was home for the summer. On balance, I thought that even though I had a low level job, which I really wasn't very good at, with very little prospects - I did at least have Jackie. The Summer holiday came and went all too quickly;

Jackie and I managed to grab a camping holiday in a wet and windy Devon (a far cry from our blissful holiday the previous year in the South of France). There was no specific thing I could point to in particular that alarmed me, but I sensed somehow that Jackie now looked on me differently. Maybe it was my own paranoia, but I imagined that as a boyfriend I must have turned out very different in reality to the proposition she had envisaged she was getting involved with. I knew she was a high achiever with big ambitions and I believed that she had begun to give up on me a little, as she was aware that I was still struggling to stay in the job at Crown Life and it was unlikely that I would ever achieve the dizzying heights she must have sought for herself and her partner. I knew I was never going to tick all of her boxes and mentally I added her name to the list of people I had disappointed. At the end of the summer, I took an additional week's holiday to help Jackie move into her new accommodation in Leeds. I remember she was very excited about having her own place for the first time, having been in halls of residence the year before, and was relishing the chance of taking her independence one step further.

I was still taking three, 400 mg tablets of lithium carbonate each day; which Google assures me is a high maintenance dosage, and whilst it was successful in stabilising my mood, I found that my emotions were being flattened and I wasn't feeling or demonstrating the same emotions towards Jackie that I had just 12 months previously (and wasn't absence meant to make the heart grow fonder?). I was quite numb, my manic elations and disabling lows had been medicated away but it seemed that the ability to feel love and demonstrate affection had been the price I had to pay for this "stability". Some years later Tim told me that he had observed when I first started taking lithium that I had become a shadow of my former self and that the spark in my character had gone. This would improve over the years as my body became more attuned to the medication, but until that equilibrium was reached the drugs I was on were taking their toll in collateral damage; they were a blunt instrument that squashed luxury items such as feelings and emotions that got in the way of doing their job. It was probably this change in my behaviour towards Jackie together with the new experiences and life style she was now enjoying as a second-year student at Leeds University which meant that our relationship, and my first love, was heading towards a close.

Jackie and I eventually came to an end at the start of the Summer of '86. It was obvious by then to both of us that we no longer felt the same way about each other as we previously had, and that our love affair was over. Not long before we ended, as I was recovering from my depression, Jackie's father had become deeply depressed and was really struggling with his life. The family surprised me as in my view, they appeared largely unsympathetic towards him. I think an affair that John had had earlier in his marriage had in truth to some extent irreparably altered the emotional loyalties in the Washington household, and he had never been completely forgiven for his past misdemeanour. To the Washingtons, John's depression appeared like another act of selfishness, and one from which he was doing nothing to make himself better. This was a far cry from the sympathy and support that the Washington family had shown to me when I was at my worst, and which undoubtedly helped me hugely in my recovery. I particularly noticed this apparent callousness in Jackie, who seemed almost indifferent to her father's illness; although I freely admit I am probably not the best person to pick up on all the subtleties and nuances of family dynamics and feelings. Then one day I received a phone call from Jackie who was distraught and in tears, saying that John had died suddenly of a heart attack. My own sympathies towards John caught me off guard and I found myself being a bit hostile towards Jackie, attacking her for what I saw as her false grief and for crying crocodile tears. I told Jackie I was surprised she was so upset since she had done nothing but complain about her father recently, and that she and her mother hadn't treated him very well in his last few months. I realise this sounds incredibly insensitive on my part (which of course it was), and indeed Jackie certainly thought so. With hindsight of course, I was totally out of order to say what I did. Can we perhaps lay the blame on my illness or the lithium? "It was the lithium talking your honour". Whatever, but at the time I felt I was seeing a side to Jackie that I had not seen before and wondering if I had misread her; Jackie was almost certainly thinking the same thing about me.

Not too long after her father had died, Jackie was at home for the summer at the end of her second year, despite the upset of her father's death she had managed to do well in her second-year exams, this was a testimony to her resilience and strength of character (a strength which I had benefitted from so much). The whole Washington family were rallying around Jackie's mother, comforting her and helping her adjust to being a widow and the responsibilities of managing her home on her own. Jackie and I were seeing each other almost daily but sadly the vital spark that had made our relationship feel so special previously, had now gone, and in truth we were going through the motions. Jackie suggested that we take a week's break from each other and feeling a bit weighed down by it all I willingly agreed that this would be a good idea. I drove her back to her mum's house and watched her go through the front door. This was the last time I ever saw her and I don't think we ever even spoke again, since I cannot remember ever discussing what was to happen after our planned one-week break. It was obvious that our separation was mutually desirable and no doubt it was a relief to both of us. Cynically speaking, the crutch and stabilising influence that Jackie had been to me, supporting me through the previous few years of crisis, had by then been replaced with something more reliable and requiring less emotional investment on my part, namely my wonder drug, Lithium.

> *It's obvious that my relationship with Jackie, my first real love, didn't end very well (what first love relationships ever do?) and I realise I had been particularly insensitive towards Jackie at a time when she needed emotional support. I am forever grateful though for Jackie coming along when I most needed someone; for all the practical and emotional support she gave me (on top of dealing with her own ordeals) the tangible results of which included helping me to acknowledge and seek help for my illness for the first time ever and giving me the encouragement and motivation to re-start my career by applying for the job with Crown Life. The rest as they say is history.*

Chapter 12 - Moving out and moving on

At least if my love life had fallen apart, other aspects of my life had become more stable. I was becoming more effective in my job and when I eventually passed my extended probationary period, I was at last made permanent and received a generous 12.5% pay rise. This was something of a major milestone for me; I had held a job down for a year, and I knew my performance was improving all the time, BUT I was still earning very little, and a 12.5% increase on fuck all is still fuck all! I had enrolled on some professional Chartered Insurance courses at Guildford College and if I passed the qualifications would look good on my CV for potential future progression. I was finding these courses quite hard going as they consisted of three hours of lectures one night a week as well as additional home study. I really struggled with my energy levels to concentrate after a taxing day at work, but with a new-found resilience and determination (surely evidence of an improved mental state) gradually I started to make progress with the exams and bit by bit aspirational thoughts of career development lodged themselves in my head.

After about two and a half years working for Crown Life, encouraged by a work colleague and good friend Steve Bolton, I changed teams and joined the Share Exchange department where Steve was a supervisor. Steve and I had got to know each other well through work and our mutual love of beer and football. Also, we had both started playing squash in a works league, which was to prove really helpful in making good business contacts. I was playing squash three or four times a week and I had started to notice that one side effect of playing this very strenuous and vigorous sport, was that through sweating profusely, I was excreting some of the lithium and this appeared to nullify some of the dulling side-effects the drug had been having on me. I felt sharper, clearer headed, and more able to process thoughts and act coherently than I had for a long time. I believe there is research out there that backs up the theory that lithium loss through sweating can be substantial and potentially even problematic if too excessive.

I was very grateful to Crown Life for the part it had played in my recovery towards a more normalised way of life. I had started picking things up far more quickly at work, no longer worrying over my mental frailties or talking to brokers. My technical knowledge of pensions and life insurance contracts had increased dramatically, to the point that I felt competent and capable in my work, a feeling that I had not experienced for many years. By February 1986, I had concluded that since the opportunities for development and promotion within Crown were limited, the only way to seriously progress my career, was to change jobs. At the time the deregulation of the UK financial system in the mid-1980s meant that the sector was booming, and lots of the larger financial institutions, including life insurance companies, were crying out for people to join them. So, it was against this backdrop and emboldened by my rediscovered motivation and ambition (yes, I was ambitious and optimistic again) that I started looking for new jobs.

The catalyst for my eventual move from Crown, was a colleague Steve Kenny and another colleague and friend, Ian. All three of us played in a works five-a-side team, and whilst enjoying a post-match pint in the pub one night, they started discussing their forthcoming career moves to companies based in London. We all wanted to live in London, particularly Ian and Steve who, being more experienced and senior than I was, were moving into well paid jobs, whereas I was content to be contemplating a move to any kind of administrative position that paid enough for me to survive in London. The recruitment agency I had registered with had succeeded in getting me an interview at Aetna Life Insurance, where through a quirk of fate it transpired that the young manager looking to recruit to his department, was an ex Crown Life employee, who had been very friendly with my boss Barry. For once in my life I seemed to be getting a break, my references held up and as on this occasion no medical history was required; to my delight I got the job. And so, it was that Steve, Ian, Paul Simpson (a friend of Steve's from Manchester) and myself, secured a tenancy on a house in Norbury in South London.

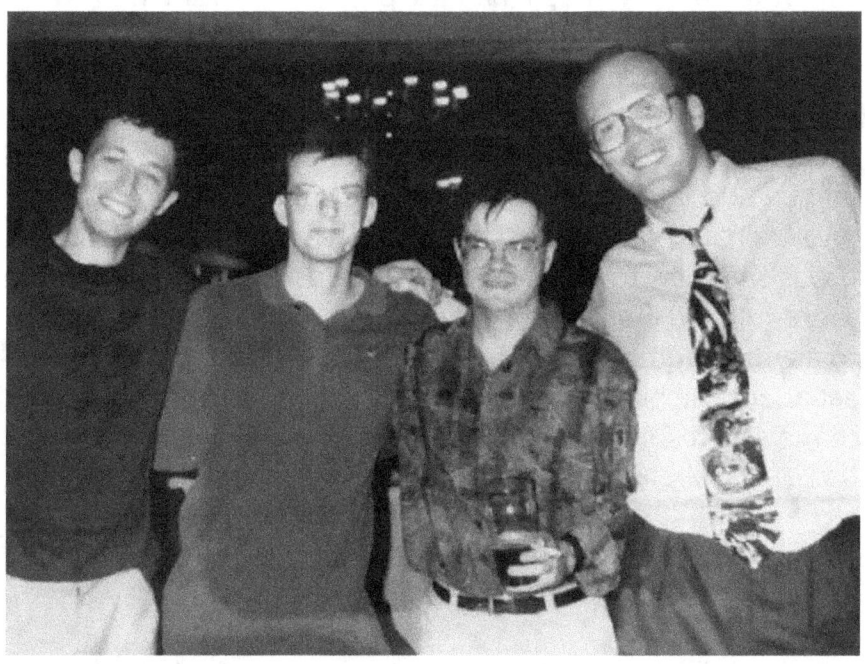

From R to L Steve, Paul Simpson, Ian and myself – the four amigos from our house in Norbury.

We moved into our new place at the beginning of July, all four of us on a high, relishing our new circumstances and the limitless prospects of living in London. Although our house was pretty ugly to look at (it was painted a violent orangey red colour), it was large enough for us to each have our own bedroom, a good-sized living room/lounge, and a small dining space to eat, just off the kitchen. We were very close to Norbury train station, a godsend as all of us needed to commute for work, and crucially, as far as I was concerned, the rent was relatively cheap. I had calculated that if I sold my car quickly and ran a tight budget I could avoid going into the red in the short term. My new job was easy to adjust to and involved issuing cheques to clients who were depositing their investment bond policies. My salary had gone from £5,600 per annum to £7,000 per annum, but of course my overheads had skyrocketed now that I had to pay for my rent and keep. Fortunately, soon after I started, increased business at work meant there were plenty of opportunities for overtime which would pay for me to have just a bit of a social life as well. Mentally I was definitely going through a purple patch; the fatigue and lethargy that had so commonly accompanied any big life changes for me before was nowhere to be seen, and so it was with new friends and a new beginning that I was living a more fulfilled life. I didn't speak about my previous problems to anyone, putting them firmly in the background and instead set about catching up on the years of fun that I felt were owed to me as a result of the time lost due to my illness.

Catch up time

Steve was a real socialite and the driving force in the house. He had a very sharp sense of humour that endeared him to other people, and consequently he always seemed to have a large network of friends and contacts. He and I were both crazy about football and shared a love for Manchester United; he a born Red Mancunian, whilst I was a Cockney red, and of course we both worked in the financial industry. Together with the others we had a great time and made a good team. Physically, Steve was a sight to behold. Whereas Paul, Ian, and I were fairly regular shaped and regular sized (maybe a little on the short side), certainly not stand out in a crowd kind of guys, Steve was the complete opposite. Standing (or more often stooping) at about six foot five inches tall, he closely resembled a praying mantis with arms and legs that looked out of proportion to the rest of his body. When I first met him, he was particularly skinny and would regularly wear a bandana, in some kind of tribute to U2! (but also, in an attempt to hide the fact that he was losing his hair, although only in his early 20s). With Steve what you saw was what you got, he maintained his limitless energy and infectious enthusiasm 24/7. I frequently found myself wondering what his mental secret was, although given that this was the 1980s and he worked in the financial sector maybe his energy was chemically enhanced (only kidding Steve).

Unsurprisingly, a couple of weeks after we had moved in, Steve suggested we should have a house warming party, which we all agreed would be a great idea. Steve largely organised it; sorting the music and putting the word around that we were having a party. Paul and I sorted the drinks and prepared the punch; an essential ingredient for any party where you want people to get pissed as quickly and as cheaply as possible. And Ian...? well I don't think Ian did much at all. During the football season Ian was rarely at home as he was an absolutely fanatical Liverpool fan, travelling from London each week to every home and away game. Steve's popularity and following, pretty much assured us of a good turnout, although I thought it unlikely that I would know many people beyond my immediate housemates. At the party a young woman that none of us knew, arrived with Linnis, one of Steve's friends. Small and wiry with a dark complexion, she had an electric energy and charisma about her which I found compelling from the minute I first set eyes on her, and so I began to ease my way over to the group she was standing with. She was obviously being very funny and all those around her were laughing out loud as she cracked joke after joke. I introduced myself and started talking with her, noting that I was a little drunk as she also appeared to be. From what I could understand she was saying through a strong Northern Irish accent, and in between frequent drags on her cigarettes, her name was Barbara, she was from Ballymena, and she was studying at Queen's University in Belfast. She had short brownish hair and a pixyish look to her and I was once again smitten and in love. Barbara was twenty, and having finished her first year at University, she had come to London for the summer to work. She was staying with Linnis and their friend Anne-Marie, also from her home town, and all of a sudden, the future, at least the short-term future, was looking incredibly rosy. Barbara and I became an item over that summer of 1986 and life with her was a rollercoaster, one which this time I was determined, I would not fall off.

Chapter 13 - Living the dream

So I was up and running in London and life seemed too good to be true. As the members of the house got to know each other better, we would regularly meet up in town after work for a few beers. The Tattershall Castle boat pub on the Thames, at Embankment, was a popular location and became our preferred meeting place as it was very easy to get to and well placed if we decided to make a night of it and go on somewhere. I always had a feeling of excited anticipation as I left my office, near The Angel Islington, with a couple of overtime hours under my belt as a financial cushion and headed into town to meet up. I was very conscious of my finances in those days and so I would stop at a couple of beers, which were a very expensive commodity in London. Also, I had learned from experience that drinking excessive amounts of alcohol did not play well with my lithium levels and could bring back symptoms of depression and problems concentrating; a double Negative. But just to meet up with friends on a warm summer's night, feeling that things were going okay, and that there were no obvious obstacles coming at me down the road was a novel and very enjoyable experience.

Nothing stays the same for long in the world of house sharing in London, and soon after having moved into the house in Norbury, Ian secured a new job back in his home city of Liverpool. This was a shame, but Ian was always the least present member of the household as most of the time he was either travelling to or from watching football matches or locked away in his room with his girlfriend. Ian was quickly replaced by a new lodger Max, the brother of Caroline, an ex-girlfriend of Ian and a colleague of Steve. That's the way it works when it comes to bloke's house sharing. I think someone had met Max, and although he was a bit younger than the rest of us, thought he was alright, would be a good fit, and most importantly would keep the flow of rent income coming in. Max had just moved from Wales to London to take up a job with National Westminster Bank as a trainee computer operator. More significant to me, although I didn't know it at the time, was that as a result of Max moving in, I would get to know his sister, Caroline, on the occasions when our social lives crossed paths. Although initially on moving into London, I had looked to Steve and Paul Simpson as the anchors of my social life I was now meeting lots of new people myself. Keith had moved to London and was living nearby, and Paul Nolan (Keith's mate from Ponty') was also in London, attempting to make it in a band. Added to this, I got to know a lot of younger Irish people through Barbara's friends and family, including her brother Michael, who's droll, laid-back sardonic sense of humour really appealed to me, and still cracks me up on the rare occasions we meet or speak on the phone these days.

My social life was quite full back then. I was still attempting to be a dutiful son to my grandparents by paying them regular visits, when if I was lucky, I would also catch up with Vernon, Chris, and Julie. I also used these visits as an opportunity to judiciously check on the state of my grandparents' house in which I now had a financial interest as my name had been added to the deeds. I remember that travelling back to Frimley Green was always a bit of a pain then, partly because I had sold my car, no longer needing one in London, and I had to make the journey by train and tube. During the hot summers weekends in those early months at Norbury, Barbara, Paul, and myself, would sometimes take the bus to Streatham common to sunbathe, together with what felt like the rest of the population of south London. I still loved laying in the sun, although Paul and Barbara with their fair complexions were less keen and would no doubt have preferred a beer and a fag in the shade of a pub close by. Towards the end of that summer, before Barbara had returned to Queen's University, the three of us, together with Paul's girlfriend, all went on holiday to the Algarve in Portugal. My only memories of that holiday are that it was extremely hot, Barbara got sun stroke (her pale Irish skin not being well suited to the climate), and consequently her face reddened and ballooned to comical proportions. Oh no, I do remember another thing; Barbara was decidedly pissed off.

By then Steve was pretty much doing his own thing; financially he was in a much healthier position than Paul and myself, and together with a friend of his, Jez, he bought a flat in East Croydon. Our six-month honeymoon period in the house had come to an end and it was all change from the original line-up. By the end of the summer, Ian had gone, Steve had gone, and Barbara (together with a fairly regular entourage of visitors from Ireland) had gone back to Belfast, leaving Paul, Max, and myself in the house. While things were still good between us, we needed a fourth lodger to bring some extra dynamism (and cash) into the house. Following notices placed in the local newsagent saying we had a room to let, there followed three fairly short-lived new lodgers in quick succession, none of whom really fitted for reasons ranging from substance addiction to renewed love affairs. So, we decided to take it a bit more seriously and we placed a proper ad' in the local newspaper, hoping that this might attract more professional and reliable types. We had a number of applicants and this time we took our time with the interviews and didn't rush to a decision. Eventually Liz, a bubbly 27-year-old Australian girl, on a year's working visa to the UK whilst on a sabbatical from her real job in a bank in Australia, came to live with us.

Despite these domestic setbacks and occasional disharmony

within the household, my career was going from strength to strength. I had got to grips with my job at Aetna insurance and was beginning to feel at ease there, when out of the blue I was contacted again by my guardian angel at the recruitment agency saying that they had seen a job opportunity that they thought would make for a good career progression for me, in the new business section of Norwich Union in Fenchurch Street. Of course, they didn't really give a toss about my career development, or at least they did only as far as their commission was concerned. I said that I thought that after only having been in my job for six months, might it not be too quick to make a change? "Au contraire", my Guardian Angel assured me (remember this was the 1980s and following deregulation the financial sector in London was struggling to meet the demand of the huge growth in jobs). She was right; I applied and was offered the job as a trainee consultant, a move which immediately increased my salary from £7,000 to £9,300, and after six months in the job I received a Union negotiated pay rise (I wasn't even in the Union) which took my salary to the giddy heights of £12,000 per annum (about £30,000 in today's money). Still not a lot in London terms, but approaching double what I had been on when I had moved there just a year previously, and far more in tune with what would have been considered a reasonable salary for someone my age. Now that I was no longer living hand to mouth, I even had enough money to go and visit Barbara and her clan in Ballymena, Northern Ireland.

Barbara, bliss, booze, and Liz

Although Barbara had gone back to Queen's University to continue with her studies, with my increased disposal income I had begun flying quite regularly to Belfast to see her for weekend visits. Barbara was living with Leo, her cousin Anne's boyfriend, who I had got to know quite well. During my visits, we would spend time drinking in the student union bar, or watching daytime TV, as Barbara and Leo followed the soaps' story lines religiously. At the end of Barbara's second year i.e., June 1988, Barbara came back to London to again work for the summer, and I was excited that she would be moving back in with me. I had had several girlfriends by then, but this was to be the first time that I felt officially in a real relationship and living with someone. We were fairly casual about "us," and planned to just see how things went and have a good time - "It'll be grand" I remember Barbara saying. Barbara resumed her job from the previous summer, selling fireplaces, and I went off each day to my job at Norwich Union, we were just like a real couple. Towards the end of the summer, we went on holiday to Malta; a trip which included two noteworthy incidents. The first was that we made friends with a British couple touring on their motorbikes around Europe. Their motorbikes, a BMW 900 and a BMW 650, were what initially attracted my interest, and having got chatting with them we had a couple of drinks and subsequently went out for a meal together. During the meal when I asked the guy, Eric, what he did for a living, he modestly replied saying he was involved in theatre and TV, and then it hit me; he was Sergeant Bob Cryer, from the TV series the Bill. Don't get too excited this exciting story ends just there. The second notable incident was that one morning I left Barbara asleep in bed and went to explore the town where we were staying. There were a lot of people milling around as it was a Sunday morning and I decided to explore one of the local churches, which were packed. As I stepped out of the bright sun and into the dark surrounds inside the church I promptly passed out. I was only briefly unconscious and got quickly to my feet unhurt but a little embarrassed as the worshippers looked at me in surprise, I made a rapid exit and walked away; what was that all about? It would happen again!

I was relieved when Barbara got her old job back selling fireplaces as it stopped her from partying quite so hard, particularly midweek. A long time ago I had met another guy from Belfast, who on one late night drinking session told me, "There's plenty of time to rest when you're in your grave." I don't think that is necessarily an Irish saying, but it is certainly a mantra which a lot of the Irish people I have met appeared to live their lives by. But I was becoming a bit concerned that all the partying, heavy drinking, and late nights might well put me in an early grave. I was being dragged along by Barbara to lots of parties and celebrations and I had begun regularly drinking large volumes of alcohol, which of course I shouldn't have been, not least because of my medication. Liz, our new Australian lodger, also turned out to be a bit of a social creature (no surprise there either) and always seemed to be able to find time for a drink. The Irish and the Australians, both being famous for their globetrotting, always seem to me to have large, constantly circulating friendship groups, and Barbara and Liz were no exception to this rule. Our household was constantly being buoyed by Barbara's friends and family over from Ireland for one reason or another, as well as a never ending stream of Liz's acquaintances on their way to or from somewhere else, or just needing to crash somewhere for a night/week or two. It was certainly a busy period with people sleeping everywhere and at one time there were about 10 people staying in the house, including a couple sleeping in a campervan parked outside the house, which was temporarily out of operation whilst being renovated for the next leg of a European tour.

A new equilibrium

My role in the broker support office at Norwich Union

presented me with a steep new learning curve, and although true to form, I started slowly, I found that after a couple of months I was able to more easily absorb information and follow the procedures and systems required in administering the new business generated by the consultants. I was now working at the sharp (sales) end of the pensions and life assurance world, and our team's success was measured exclusively by how much business the consultants could generate and how quickly we could process the resulting paperwork. This role gave me a much deeper understanding and familiarity with how things worked at Norwich Union, including close knowledge across the breadth of their products. My new job title was Trainee Consultant and my aim was that at some point, when I was ready, I would apply to become a consultant myself, thereby contributing to the generation of new business which would ensure all my office-based colleagues were kept busy and got paid at the end of the month. At first, I found my relationships with these colleagues a bit strained; I am certain that my shortcomings were all too apparent to the experienced and knowledgeable office staff, who must have been thinking that if their future bonuses were dependent upon my success, then they would surely go hungry. This attitude did change over time as I got better at my job, although no doubt I did give them plenty of reason at the beginning to justify their early apprehensiveness and coldness towards me.

However, I persisted, and as with all my previous jobs, when I settled down and felt less stressed, my anxieties lessened, and my mind responded by enabling me to take on board and retain more detailed information (detail was king in that world) and contribute (and importantly be seen to contribute) towards the team's productivity. Little by little as my skills, knowledge, and productivity improved, I established myself as an integral part of the back up support team to our consultants,

Harry and Rob. I worked tirelessly to become an expert in the world of pensions and to keep up to date with the ever-changing legislation that determined the what's, the why's, and the how's of everything we did. At that time Norwich Union had continued to offer "with profits" policies, which were a safe and good investment, particularly as the market emerged from the economic crash of 1987 and consequently Norwich Union was thriving as a business.

Summer of '89

By the summer of 1989 I had reached the end of my training, and I was therefore, at least in theory, ready to go on to the final stage of the selection process to become a Norwich Union consultant (this had become a dream goal for me). Under normal circumstances, for trainees having completed their training, this was largely a formality and a foregone conclusion. The selection process itself being that the aspiring consultants (of which there were 12 on this occasion), myself included, would deliver a presentation to a panel at our Billericay offices. With the knowledge, skills, and experience I had gained in the 18 months since I had been at Norwich Union, I was technically more than capable of this task, ...and here comes the but..., BUT still not fully appreciating the delicate relationship between my state of mind and my medication regime, two weeks before the selection event I took the unilateral decision to temporarily come off my lithium in the lead up to the interview. My naïve thinking was that this strategy would help un-fog my mind, thus providing me with additional clarity and energy to ensure I gave a presentation that fully demonstrated my competence and suitability for the role of a full consultant. You will probably have spotted the flaw in my thinking and may even be ahead of me in imagining the consequences of my poor decision making. Maybe, just maybe, I could have scraped through had I prepared sufficiently and at least had this to fall back on; but of course, I hadn't.

I knew I was nervous and agitated during my presentation but judging by the laughter and amusement on the faces of the panel members, I gauged that things were going quite well and that the panel members were on my side as I took them comprehensively, if a little haphazardly, through the benefits of a flexible "whole of life" policy. About a week later, now securely back on my meds in line with my crafty plan, my manager called me into his office and told me that I had not been successful at the panel and would not be confirmed as a full consultant. As part of his feedback, more powerful and devastating than any verbal feedback could have been, he showed me a video recording of my presentation. What I saw nearly broke me on the spot. What I observed was not me giving a presentation, in any recognisable sense of the word, instead I witnessed a person, resembling me, making incomprehensible, incoherent, manic utterances, as those of a crazed lunatic. What I had mistaken at the time as supportive, encouraging laughter from the panel members, I now understood was in fact barely controlled hilarity as they watched on in amazement as the circus came to town. I wouldn't have trusted the man in that video to sell popcorn in a cinema let alone to get the trust of brokers to sell lifetime investment products and policies to businesses. The one saving grace in the feedback was that I was told I could continue doing the sales support office-based work I had been doing and in which I had demonstrated my competence; I anticipated a change in my job title though.

It is a well-documented problem that many patients suffering with mental illness will at different times, and of their own volition without consultation with their GP, vary, skip or stop

> *taking their meds. The reasons for this are varied and very individual but include; wanting relief from the numbness of emotions, inability to think clearly, unpleasant side effects, perhaps their condition itself. Research shows that the sudden stopping of taking lithium can have disastrous effects for the patient including "rebound" which is a rapid onset and worsening of the bipolar symptoms.*

Strangely this disastrous experience, rather than dampening my enthusiasm to become a consultant, actually fired me on. I knew from my role in the sales office at Norwich Union, that I had gained vital insight into what was required to be a successful consultant including, product knowledge, an understanding of broker motivation, and the role of the sales team in supporting the effective consultant. Whilst my presentation style had undoubtedly been idiosyncratic, I took some confidence in the skills and knowledge I had acquired, which had demystified for me, the once hallowed role of the consultant. For this reason and my intuition that my future as a consultant with Norwich Union was now gone forever, I decided that I should seize the day and immediately apply for consultant positions outside of Norwich Union. Fortunately for me, insurance companies were still looking to expand their operations and after one long, this time appropriately medicated interview, I was offered the job as a consultant with Prolific Life Insurance company; my reward for my boldness being an increase in my basic pay, a company car, and a mortgage subsidy worth £2,400 per year. Of course, the added appeal of the consultant role, and the Holy Grail to any sales job in the pensions sector was the opportunity to earn commission on top of my basic salary; if of course and it was a big IF, I could reach what appeared to be patently unrealistic and unrealisable sales targets, which in retrospect, they proved to be.

Thankfully the wobble following my meddling with my medication did not result in any lasting upsets to my mental wellbeing, and once again I found myself entering the summer on a high with a new job and with new prospects. It felt like this was just the lift I needed to move towards the next stage of my life, although I didn't underestimate the size of the challenge. Prolific was a small insurance company and my patch was to be South-East London; a big area and one in which I inherited no existing key accounts that I could upsell to. I was in essence a development consultant, seeking to bring in new business in a new patch from scratch. Despite assurances when I started the job that I would be given a database of warm broker contacts, these never materialised, and I found myself looking up brokers from the listings in the Yellow Pages. In truth Prolific's products were not that well known and also they were not overly attractive to brokers. The company had done pretty well in the past and some of the Unit Trust Funds had performed outstandingly in the early 1980s, but since 1987 they had on the whole performed miserably. My only hope lay in my ability to present the statistics on our products performance in a way that made them look most positive - as Frank Carson used to say, "it's the way you tell them". Well, I had my own Frank Carson to help me, he came in the form of my colleague and trainer/mentor, Brian, an ex-building Society manager, who was a great salesman and who I learned a lot from shadowing for my first couple of months. I began putting into practice the approaches I had seen Brian demonstrate and coupled with some good marketing angles provided by Prolific, this helped me get my feet inside the front door of a number of brokers. Although these appointments gave me some respite with my bosses, they didn't generate any sales, and I soon realised that getting to see brokers was going to be the easy part of the job. I was incredibly busy, working very hard and seeing lots of people (and lots of South London) but I wasn't generating any new business.

My travels around my patch were at least being made more enjoyable by the new company car I was driving around in. It was a Ford Fiesta XR2; a boy racer car if ever there was one. Within 48 hours of having taken possession of the car I had crashed it, my fault entirely. No one was hurt but the car was destined for the repair shop where it remained for the next four weeks. When it came back, I was back on the road but after only another two weeks I had pranged it again; this time reversing at speed into a streetlamp. At this point my manager Richie had a word with me stating in no uncertain terms that if I crashed the car one more time, I would be history. He probably viewed this as an opportunity for them to cut their losses as I wasn't much of an asset to them at the time and still hadn't brought in any new business. In addition to this latter point, Richie had received a few negative reports about me from some of my brokers, saying that I didn't know enough about the subject I was talking about and I was beginning to appear like a bit of a liability as far as my reputational balance sheet at Prolific was concerned. It was under these conditions that Richie arranged to come out with me and observe first-hand how I performed in front of the brokers. By the time he did actually come out with me though I was a lot more up to speed on the subject of small, self-administered pension schemes (yawn!) and I put on a good show in front of him. I believed that the problem was more with the brokers I was seeing, as they were not specialists and were used to mainly selling bread and butter products, which were not in the portfolio of products Prolific had to offer. Often the criticisms from the brokers related to previous Prolific products they had sold, in which had seen the value of their clients' policies go down. My apparent weakness was in not appearing confident in front of these brokers when attempting to defend the indefensible i.e., the more recent track record of these Prolific schemes.

The visits with Richie had gone well; I had measured up and demonstrated my skills as a consultant, as well as my product knowledge, and Richie saw me give a good account of myself in front of the brokers. Another month passed and I was still in the job; not only that, I was starting to generate some business. My first success is worth mentioning as it illustrates the creativity and adaptability that was required from me to get an in to bring in new business to Prolific at that time, and one in which I had doggedly risen to the challenge. Ultimately it was a numbers game and if you kissed enough frogs then you got to meet the Princess sooner or later. On my first deal, once again sourced from the yellow pages, I had obtained the home address of a registered broker in West Wickham, and unannounced, I stopped at his expensive looking house. The guy stressed to me that he only really sold policies for his family, which was the only reason he was registered as a broker (this type of small-scale operation was not untypical of the brokers I found myself working with), and all his pensions business went through his swimming pool company! To cut a long story short we ended up in his back garden sitting by his pool (drinking a beer) and he told me about two of his business partners who were going into a new risky line of business and would require massive life insurance cover. I walked away from that house being able to write three £1 million contracts and the broker got a great deal on his commission. The other successful outcome which came from that speculative, chance visit was that my job was safe for a little while longer.

In my wonderfully sporty white XR2, I drove down to see my grandparents every couple of weeks. My grandfather's health had deteriorated quite significantly, he had lost some weight and was looking a bit frail; but all things considered he wasn't doing too badly for a man approaching 80. Also, these short breaks provided some respite from the noisy environment of my house in Norbury, although it did mean subjecting myself again to my grandmother's discordant but familiar tantrums. The longer I lived away from Frimley Green, the more I enjoyed coming back to my hometown, I began to see the place I once took for granted from a totally new perspective. Enough time and distance had passed to allow me to remember the good times I had there as a child, and it felt great to visit on my terms rather than running to it as somewhere to hide away following my most recent breakdown, such as after my disastrous experiences at Kent University and Thames Polytechnic.

Chapter 14 - An early sign of trouble

Back in London as we moved towards the height of summer, the partying became more frantic, and Barbara became louder and more argumentative than ever; particularly on the occasions when we met up with her brothers, Michael, and Arthur in London. By this time Barbara had converted me to smoking, a habit I had always been disgusted by in my youth and my memories of the constant blue plume of cigarette smoke that had hung around our front room from my grandfather's and Uncle Peter's non-stop chain smoking. As if this wasn't bad enough, Barbara had also introduced me to smoking dope, which I only did occasionally and in strict moderation out of some sense of self-preservation of my mental health. Despite my considerable alcohol consumption, which often included lunch time entertaining with my brokers, I had kept myself reasonably fit through playing squash, running, weights exercise etc. I was beginning to feel (and look) like one of those footballers from the 1970s, who combined a debauched lifestyle of drinking and smoking alongside exhausting training sessions and matches; they appeared pretty healthy to the casual observer but were abusing their bodies every which way. You certainly couldn't get away with that lifestyle in the modern game and I suspect the same goes for the world of insurance and pensions consultants – it's nothing up the nose, apart from a hanky or a Vicks vapo rub inhaler.

One summer evening, Barbara, her cousin Anne, and I were on the night bus returning to Norbury after a night out at a pub in

Streatham. Normally whenever travelling on double decker buses at night around Brixton/Streatham, I preferred to sit downstairs, it just felt the sensible option in an area of London that could sometimes resemble more a wild west frontier town than a London suburb. On this particular occasion, Barbara and Anne, both the worse for drink, insisted on going upstairs so that Barbara could have a cigarette out of sight of the driver. As well as the three of us and another lone traveller quietly reading his newspaper, there were three other young guys at the back of the top deck of the bus. It was obvious that these three were having a good night as they were being quite loud and boisterous; on any other night, under these circumstances, this would have been my cue to go back to the safety of the lower deck.

One of the guys, dripping with gold jewellery and sporting a gold front tooth, came up to us and aggressively demanded a cigarette from Barbara who had by then already lit herself one up. Now, if there existed a set of rules that you should live your life by, I am sure that, "don't demand a cigarette from a drunk girl from Belfast" would be on the list. So, it was not surprising that in reply to the guys less than courteous request, Barbara told him to "feck off". After that, things developed quite quickly. I was just about to suggest to Barbara, that in everyone's interest maybe she could see her way to giving the guy a fag after all, but she proceeded to render this potential goodwill offer a non-starter, by letting forth a stream of abuse towards the young man. He, not being suitably eloquently equipped to enter into Socratic debate with this Irish banshee, instead responded physically and lashed out punching Barbara in the face. "Fuck"! I thought, "now I've got to do something, or I'll never hear the end of it"; at the same time as noticing that we were pulling up at our stop. Instinctively I stood up and laid into our aggressor with a volley of punches to his head, several of which I could feel had landed well. At this point I was overran by his two pals and somehow, I managed to shuffle into a defensive position under a seat at the front of the bus, as all three of them returned fire I still had enough wits about me to protect my face and ward off a few of the blows they were throwing. The bus driver hearing the screams had stopped the bus and was now shouting from downstairs. At the sound of his shouts both Barbara and Anne ran down the stairs followed by the three guys, leaving me curled up under the front seats but completely unscathed. I got up and ran downstairs weighing up my next move just as one of the three threw a parting punch at Anne, hitting her square in the jaw. Barbara and I then turned our attention towards Anne who was now truly hysterical having experienced up close and personal the highs and the lows of a London night out. I think Barbara was somewhat chastened, as she realised that if she had given the guy a cigarette this could have all turned out differently, we might even have become friends, and Anne might have avoided her punch in the face. As the bus pulled away, I glanced up at the top deck and saw the other passenger still sitting there deeply engrossed in his newspaper, oblivious or uncaring to what had just happened- I grudgingly admired his tactic.

Take from this experience any lessons that you can, but let me also suggest a few of my own for your benefit; don't travel on the top deck of a night bus in London at midnight if you can avoid it, a little generosity with your smokes when demanded by a group of drunk lads although distasteful might be well be the better course of action, and confrontation is not always the best form of defence. Afterwards, Barbara claimed that these would be her preferred course of action if she ever found herself in a similar position again, although whether she would follow her own advice is something that I hoped she would never have to find out. After a few minutes' recovery time, we got off the bus and thankfully the three guys were nowhere to be seen. Good job, as I don't think my fighting skills would have been sufficient to defend us out in the open and under different circumstances. We were lucky to walk away from this situation physically relatively unscathed, although we were all quite shaken up. I have often thought how fortunate we had been that night and how things could have gone differently. What if I had been wearing my glasses and not my contact lenses? What if any of our assailants had been carrying a knife? (seemingly a mandatory item of apparel these days) and also how little impact my salvo of punches seemed to have had on our attackers. My blurred memories of golden-tooth and his scarred face made me think that he was no stranger to violence, and that we had indeed all got away lightly.

Approximately six weeks after the bus incident, my body and mind were telling me that things needed to ease up or else I was headed for trouble. I knew that I could no longer keep up such a hectic home and social life and continue to be effective at work. The regular late-night midweek drinking sessions with Barbara, Paul, and Max and our extended Irish and Australian household members, were taking a serious toll on me. What they did was up to them but from that point onwards I started going to bed early (if you call midnight early), leaving Barbara still smoking and drinking with the others. I had come to realise that it would be better for me to split up with Barbara; it had been a great adventure, full of laughs and good memories, but she would soon return to Belfast for her third year and in all honesty, I no longer felt the same way about her. Eventually everything came to a head one Saturday morning in the middle of an angry argument, after which Barbara immediately left the house on bad terms, the few possessions she had with her in London, packed into a rucksack as she headed towards Michael's place in Clapham.

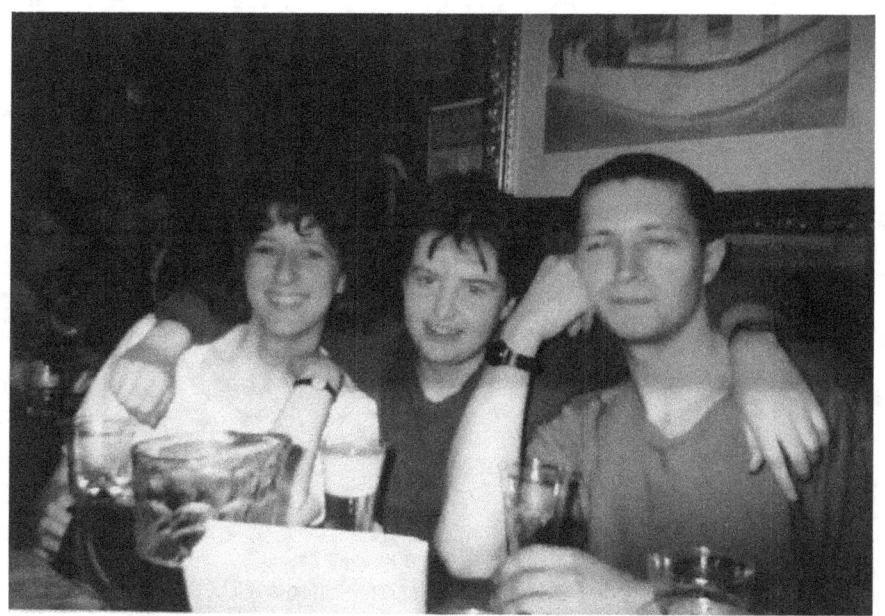

Me together with Barbara (middle) and Laura (Michael's wife) – unsurprisingly in a pub.

Young, free & single

Following Barbara's dramatic and sudden departure, life became a lot calmer as the partying and shouting stopped and I found things far more moderate and calmer in most aspects of my daily life. This had additional immediate benefits as it reduced my stress levels and I refocussed, ensuring that I did not put myself under excessive pressure either at work or in my social life; instead, my goal became to live and work within my comfort zone and at all costs maintain my stability. Having adapted to my new single status and confident in my work, I saw this period as an opportunity to invest in the quality rather than the quantity of my social life; and to better enjoy the richness of those relationships with a small circle of close friends. Now that Liz the Aussie had also moved on, the population of our house was much reduced with just Paul, Max, and myself living there. Although Steve had moved back to Altringham, we re-kindled our friendship and about the same time I got to know Pat one of my brokers a lot better. Pat and I got on really well, and I am pleased to say that we became lifetime friends. Later in my life, I struck up a good friendship with his son Ryan as well, when he came to stay with me after I had moved to Poland and before he started university.

Confidence is the key

I am sure that anyone who has ever suffered with depression will know that feeling confident and secure in your sense of self, can take a long time to achieve but it can disappear in the blink of an eye; to be replaced with uncertainty, self-doubt, insecurity, and crushing anxiety. So what I was doing at that time was almost a textbook exercise in attempting to compartmentalise and manage my life. I was trying to do this through a multi-pronged strategy i.e. (i) controlling my work life and avoiding work related stress whenever I could; (ii) enjoying my social life and the company of others but within a boundaried approach (iii) laying down some firm pragmatic foundations by developing a financial future; (iv) and significantly, taking a break from the complications of an emotional relationship (not least as I had my work cut out already with the other three priorities I was striving for).

This was a rewarding period for me practically and emotionally, and I felt mentally strong and at ease with myself. I remember a play I been to see called Melon, at the theatre in Guildford. In Melon, the main character was a guy whose life had come off the rails. He had completely lost his moral compass, he had cheated on his wife, was a heavy drinker, and ultimately lost his business – resulting in him having a nervous breakdown. The play showed how Melon started to help his own recovery by acknowledging his downfall and becoming aware of the need to tread carefully in life. Taking small deliberate steps and avoiding the false appeal of things that would invariably bring stress and failure, pursuing instead the more ordinary and mundane but ultimately more fulfilling and self-actualising things in life. Melon had only learned this lesson by having personally experienced the pitfalls of living the opposite lifestyle. I think that, at that time, similar to Melon I had learned at first hand, how within the context of my bipolar condition, that although I would never be immune to the mania and depression that the illness brought with it, I could potentially manage my way through the extreme consequences of my illness through constant vigilance and awareness of my vulnerabilities and mitigating them through my lifestyle choices. Unfortunately it proved to be far easier to convince myself of this more pedestrian but rewarding way of living when I was calm and rational, than it was for me follow the same advice when I was in the middle of manic phase of my illness as we shall soon see.

1990

By now, the general trajectory of my professional life was definitely upwards. I was consistently feeling mentally stronger, less chaotic, and more optimistic about life; furthermore, I had learned from my past experiences, and I was more disciplined in my monitoring and self-maintenance, and I was careful not to let the daily disciplines and routines that were crucial to managing my wellbeing slip. I tried to move forward in small, controlled steps rather than leaps and bounds, which could take me precipitously close to the edge of the abyss. In pursuit of this greater sense of self determination and security, I decided that the time had come for me to move out of rented accommodation, and with the purchasing power of my new income (and perhaps some overly generous mortgage lending ratio's by the banks) I bought a flat in South Croydon, which I hoped would remove me forever from the whims of the private rented sector. Ironically this turned out to be just about the worst financial decision I have ever made, but at the time, it made sense. I took my own lodger, Paul Simpson, with me, which guaranteed me an additional line of income to help offset some of the cost of the mortgage repayments. Yes, looking back it was a poor financial decision to buy into that market at that time as house price value dropped by about 18% in the crash of 1990, however at the time I did at least feel more secure as a property owner (and landlord).

I suspect I have been slightly gilding the lily when I talk about my newfound disciplined approach to life, one in which I was careful not to repeat my past mistakes. On some level, I must have felt that ending with Barbara was a mistake, because about six months after we had finished, I went to Belfast to attempt a reunion. This feeling was short lived however, and it was obvious when I got there that Barbara had moved on emotionally and romantically and was already going out with an old flame of hers. Good for her! And this was probably the best outcome for me as I am sure that it would not have been healthy for me to go back into that frenetic exhausting relationship. I learned a couple of hard lessons from this experience: "the grass is always greener on the other side" and "once you lose something or someone that you took for granted you can never get them back". So it was, I returned to South Croydon, wiser and reflective, but still upbeat. Yes, I was on my own relationship wise, but I had my own place, I had a lodger to contribute towards the mortgage, I had a group of close friends who provided a good social network, and of course I had a good job that I was doing well in. I had a stable platform from which to move on from; life was good, seize the day! Make hay whilst the sun shines etc, and then completely out of the blue, I was made redundant.

Redundancy

I like to think that I didn't lose my job through any fault of my own, but that instead it was purely down to the fact that Prolific had been taken over by another company and, as one of the last in, I was one of the first out when the inevitable post-merger workforce rationalising took place. I found myself suddenly unemployed and with just one month's salary in the bank from my payoff. I needed to find another job quickly since money was tight, and on top of my mortgage repayments, I was repaying a loan to my grandmother, who had lent me £10,000 from the sale of her house in Frimley Green towards the deposit on my flat. Having borrowed the money from my grandmother, I had found myself elevated to a fast-track repayment programme, since following my grandfather's death (at last Sonny was finally getting some peace) my grandmother was going through the balance of her funds at an alarmingly rapid rate, mainly as a consequence of all the holidays she was going on which were being organised by the Church. Fortunately, by that time, I had developed a number of good professional contacts and a reasonable reputation with several of my brokers, several of whom were willing to act as referees for me. By working these networks hard, within only a couple of weeks I had secured a new job with Standard Life, a large life assurance company. Ironically the position I was offered was as a consultant, the very role I had failed to get following my disastrous presentation following the Norwich

Union assessment. There was one small hurdle that I had to overcome before the offer was made final, this was a full medical health history check. Unlike all my previous jobs where I had been able to skate over the details around my chequered mental health, Standard Life wanted a far more detailed report, in part because I would be joining their employee pension scheme, which included quite a lot of life insurance cover.

Anyone who has a hidden health condition or a disability lives in fear of such occupational health assessments. To get to this stage in the recruitment process and then to be unsuccessful because of a previous or current, undisclosed illness, would be devastating. And of course, back in the unenlightened early 1990s, employer's fears and lack of understanding of mental illness meant that they were not inclined to look favourably on someone with a history of mental ill health, regardless of whether they were currently ill or the actual impact of their illness to their functioning. Again however, fortunately for me, over the years and many visits, I had developed quite a good relationship with my GP, who I saw every three months or so for the renewal of my repeat prescriptions. I managed to persuade her to complete the form in such a way that there was sufficient ambiguity around my treatment of depression so that it looked as if it related only to the period when my mother had died twelve years previously. I think my doctor summarised the health check by saying that I was a fit, young man who was unlikely to die in the near future, or at least during my employment at Standard Life, which is of course all they were really concerned about. And so it was, I finally achieved my goal of being a consultant, and what's more with a market leader firm Standard Life.

Chapter 15 - The next few years

By now, I had almost come to believe that there was a benevolent God looking down on me, putting things right when they went wrong and of course when I fucked up. A God, who in addition to my guardian angels at the employment agency, took an active interest in my career and who made me feel protected and looked after. Following my redundancy, which had been a real career low point, I had stepped out of the Prolific frying pan into what could best be described as a warm duvet at Standard Life. Standard Life was a much better known and more respected organisation, whose products were immensely more appealing and virtually sold themselves. This meant that I no longer had first to win over my brokers belief in me in order to then convince them to have confidence in the policies I wanted them to sell. For the first time in my career, I found myself in the novel position whereby my brokers were actually pleased to see me when I was introduced to them as the new consultant for the area. And to boot, as well as working in a sales environment that was far more conducive to my wellbeing, I was receiving a better salary, a decent level of commission, and a more secure mortgage. I still had the odd wobble when under pressure, but I had enough energy and resilience to deal with these and pass them off largely unnoticed. This new much more favourable set of circumstances relieved the work pressure on me considerably and left me freer to focus on establishing a work life balance by putting a bit more effort into sorting out my social life.

Football: here we go, here we go, here we go... again

I will endeavour to avoid becoming overly nostalgic or self-indulgent here, but I was about to experience a bit of a renaissance and at the same time reach a pinnacle in my footballing career (although of course I use the word career loosely). I think it is worthwhile devoting a bit of space to this social/leisure activity, which became so important to me, not only because I took so much enjoyment from the innate pleasure and exercise, I received from playing the "beautiful game," but also for what it provided for me in terms of its benefits to my mental health. It is now widely acknowledged that physical exercise, particularly that taken outdoors, can provide immense psychological health benefits. Its positive impacts on stress and depression levels, blood flow to the brain, improved sleep, muscle maintenance, increased vitamin D, reduced hypertension, lower levels of obesity, etc etc etc are well documented and backed up by hard science. But equally as valuable to me as the satisfaction gained by dropping a shoulder and gliding past a defender, or a well-timed anticipatory run from the midfield, or of course a firmly struck volley into the top corner (all of which I was capable of occasionally) was the camaraderie and sense of place and belonging that I experienced from playing this team sport at that particular time.

Through Brendan, a colleague at Standard Life, I was welcomed into West Wickham FC, who played in the Southern Amateur Leagues. My football skills were ropey and rusty but thanks largely to regular jogging and squash, my fitness levels were not far off what was needed to play in the lower leagues. I joined at the same time as another Standard Life colleague, Paul Healey, and in my first season there I was given the nickname "headless". This was because of my tendency to habitually run around in circles, not really knowing what to do with the ball when I got it, just as likely to score in our own goal as in the oppositions, and in reality, equally unlikely to score at either end. But after a couple of seasons, having honed what talent I had and having learned to read and understand the game better, I became a regular team selection, alongside Paul in the club's fourth team. This level suited me just fine since as with other aspects of my life, I was well aware of my limitations. I worked hard at my football and trained regularly, including throughout the closed season; and as a by-product, I became good friends with Brendan and Paul (friendships I still value to this day). I began to live for my football, the overall crack of it leaked into and enriched all aspects of my life no end. Physically, socially, mentally, in terms of personal achievement and my sense of being part of something bigger than myself; there seemed to be no limits to the benefits that being a player for West Wickham provided for me at the time. I had found a kind of family, where I was accepted and had a place and a purpose. The clubhouse banter after the game, when we would humorously dissect the match just played, including our individual contributions to it, was as enjoyable (and on occasions more so) than the game itself. I learned to love and happily accept my nickname for what it was, a familiarity and a term of affection. I don't think this communal/social aspect of team sports has been explored or analysed as much as the more direct benefits related to the exercise aspect itself; for me it wasn't just the icing on the cake, it became the cake itself; and, hey, the exercise and the endorphins could do their own thing as well.

On the work front, things remained consistently good at Standard Life, I was making progress of a sort within the company, but my biggest weakness and the one drawback which stopped me from really flying was my continued inability to stand up and give a coherent, confident, and convincing group presentation. The result was that I was unable to stand out and make a telling impression on my regional manager or other key external stakeholders, i.e., the people who could play a crucial part in my career progression. Generally though, I met my performance targets and with my ever-increasing technical knowledge and expertise, particularly in the field of pensions, I was able to generate considerable business, albeit it from existing brokers through their business churn. I wasn't setting the pensions world on fire by generating brand new business with new brokers and clients, but I knew that I was not alone in this modus operandi; as I mentioned earlier, I had learned my trade from the best.

So, my work life was ticking along nicely, my football mates and my close friends were largely meeting my social needs; what did I need to make things complete? ...ah yes, it was time to turn my attention again to my recently neglected love life. In the days before the internet, social media, and dating websites, you had to physically go out and meet people if you were looking for romance and the possibility of finding love. Invariably this meant hitting the nightclubs and bars, since this was where, if you were lucky, and/or skilled, you could "get off," with someone, as we used to say back in the 80s. No doubt today's online dating is fraught with its own risks and weaknesses, but if we can assume, for a minute, in the case of genuine, honest online punters looking for romance (a big "if" I know), they use fancy algorithms to do the leg work of eliminating, matching, and filtering you towards people who theoretically you should have things in common with and shared interests. Then, via the miracle of online chat and messaging, you can get some feedback from the virtual exchanges (again assuming we are talking about honest, genuine, non-psychopathic, financially sound people) through a deeper dive to decide whether there is sufficient interest and common ground for you to take things further i.e., to actually meet up and possibly get off with each other. This is the try before you buy approach.

The night club scenario from my experience, provides almost the complete opposite environment, and therefore requires an entirely different, more direct approach. I should say here that the Swan in Stockwell, was our preferred haunt; it was a no nonsense, down to earth club, which played a lot of Irish music, sold relatively cheap beer, didn't charge for entrance before 10pm, and offered free sausage and chips to all; in short, my kind of club[8]. Already fuelled on alcohol before going to the club, on arrival we would quickly get down to the business of sizing up the talent and planning our approach. I selected my quarry based on a traditional and flexible descending checklist of criteria, namely, was she attractive? ...was she not unattractive? ...did she smile back when I smiled at her? ...did she at least not show signs of disgust when I smiled at her? ...and finally, did she have a mate (always got to remember Paul)? Having gone through the process of applying these algorithms of my own, to help filter and fine tune my selection, I would proceed to make my move. Usually this involved asking the target to dance, or sometimes simply inserting myself into the conversation that the unexpecting young woman was at the time engaged in (this was a riskier tactic as it required that as a minimum, I needed to come up with a more scintillating line of chat than that which I had butted into). Don't get me wrong, my approach was not fool proof, and it sometimes didn't turn out well; in fact, it frequently didn't work at all, and in these instances the woman in question would make it supremely clear to me, that she was not now and never would be interested, and would I kindly just FUCK OFF!

---

[8] A recent search on the web reveals that the Stockwell Swan is still going strong and the on-line images suggest that it has lost none of its charm or sophistication.

But here comes the kicker, I was by profession an insurance salesman and I was used to knockbacks. All knockbacks were treated as an independent response to a singular event and had no bearing on the outcome of my next attempt. What's more I didn't ever stop at single events. Any salesman worth their salt, knows that bringing home the deal is a numbers game; so if a girl showed no interest in my advances, I would not let myself be disillusioned, instead I would move on to the next one; perhaps to her mate, or to her mate's mate, or to the slightly less attractive/slightly more unattractive girl standing next to them. The more I rolled the dice, the more I ensured that the odds worked in my favour; and the laws of probability told me that if I kept on trying, sooner or later someone would relent and give in, and then I would be away. Sometimes in the Swan, you would see some really ugly bloke getting off with a really attractive woman, I held these guys in awe and looked up to them in admiration since clearly, they were the best salesman in the place. They were never disheartened by rejection, they kept to their plan; they knew that the product they were pitching was subprime, but they also knew how to play the numbers game because they had done the math! Those guys could have sold Prolific policies standing on their heads. Of course, they may also have had a Porsche or a Ferrari parked outside to bolster their appeal, but in my mind that meant their success extended to their professional lives as well.

It was on the whole all good and innocent fun, and it worked because the overwhelming majority of the people going to clubs, male and female, were there for the same reason – to get lucky; after all, if you were already partnered up, why would you go to a club? Surely it would be like taking coal to Newcastle. Anyway, as a game plan, my rather unsubtle method worked well for me, so much so that sometimes it felt as if my success lay more in making sure I didn't give a girl I had approached, any reason not to get off with me. As a consequence, I often found myself going home with someone I had met only hours before.

BUT, the last thing this approach to coupling up was effective at, was as a solid basis for determining the likelihood of any successful longer-term relationship; my algorithms were written purely on the basis of achieving a much shorter-term end goal. The club environment actively worked against getting to know anything really about the other person, if that had indeed been your goal. The deafening noise virtually guaranteed that you would not have been able to hear what each other was saying, and you had to rely more on body language for communication; added to this, alcohol invariably played a big part in the mutual attraction but could also mask what the person was really like and would inevitably have worn off some hours later. The morning after such encounters could be acutely awkward upon waking in a stranger's home and bed. Frequently hasty arrangements were made for a subsequent meet up, more as part of an exit strategy to get out of the house, rather than with any real intention of following through on these plans. And on the occasions when I did meet up with a girl again, it could be quite depressing to find that the chemistry we had experienced, had been temporary, illusory and alcohol fuelled, that we had little in common, and no desire to see each other again let alone start a relationship.

I think that about sums up the highs and the lows of the experiences I had at the Swan, or enough at least to give you a general impression of my courting behaviours at the time. I am conscious that I am reporting this from my exclusively male perspective and that women may have had a different take on their Swan experiences. But I did meet and "get off with" (sorry for the language!) a number of women at the Swan, and if we assume that they were a reasonably representative sample, they appeared on the whole just as invested in that particular approach to getting together as I was. And of course, in the interest of balance I should add that many of these women, when sobered up the following morning, were just as keen to see me leave as I was to depart. Finally, in case I have painted too shallow and sordid a picture of my clubbing approach to romance, I will add that although I realised this very random approach to dating was unlikely to prove successful in realising a long term, loving, mutually respectful relationship; it was good fun and thrilling at the time, and so despite its obvious shortcomings and my reservations, I gave it a good go and so it seemed did most other people who were out clubbing as well.

Chapter 16 – Loving life, generally

Settling down, getting married

By December 1993, I could no longer kid myself that in pursuing me hedonistic social life I was still making up for the lost years of my early twenties when I struggled with my illness, and I was becoming bored and tired with my clubbing lifestyle. I wanted to move on with my life and I was looking for a more meaningful and lasting relationship. You may remember that I mentioned earlier a woman called Caroline, Max's sister, and one of Steve's old work colleagues. Well, about the same time that I was becoming disenchanted with my weekly visits to the Swan, I bumped into Caroline again at a mutual friend's Christmas party. We talked all evening and I told her that I liked her a lot and always had, ever since we had first met all those years before. This was very true, and I was shocked by just how strong my feelings were towards Caroline, and how they came tumbling out of my mouth as I told her honestly how I felt. Caroline was more muted in her response to my overtures, in part I believe as she was kind of in an existing relationship, and also because she had been given the quite justifiable impression from Steve and Max, that I was high risk when it came to relationships and commitment levels. During our semi-intimate conversation at the party, I was very truthful about my past and shared my most private thoughts with her, which I think showed her a side of me she had not been aware of; she must have liked what she saw (you see I could adapt my game plan to the circumstances).

To my amazement and delight, Caroline and I started seeing each other and in a relatively short and wonderful period of time our relationship turned into something much bigger and stronger, leading to us getting married in September 1994. We both rented out our respective flats moved into a jointly rented place in Sydenham, in South London. I brought one additional piece of baggage with me from my flat in Croydon, my new lodger Rick (Rick had replaced Paul Simpson as my lodger when Paul went off to Bruno in the Czech Republic to teach English some years earlier). As ever I welcomed the opportunity to defray some of our living costs elsewhere! After we had been married for only a few short and passionate months, we decided that we wanted to set about starting a family immediately, and as such we threw all contraception to one side and continued with our passion. Both on good salaries and having secured a high mortgage offer, we started looking for a place of our own from which to base the new family we were working hard at starting; I was confident that we would have quick success on this front since we were certainly taking it seriously and putting the hours in. Within weeks we found and put an offer in on an end of terrace house in Bromley, only a five-minute walk from the town centre. At this point, Rick moved on into a place of his own, only a couple of miles away. I liked Rick a lot, he was a very laid-back guy, however he worked ridiculously long hours at his job in the print industry and I never saw him much, even when we lived together, and when he moved out, I saw him even less.

Lo and behold practice made perfect, and before we knew it Caroline was pregnant and expecting our first, and only child together. Caroline's mother, Marylyn, had moved to Egypt a few years previously and soon after we married, we took a trip out to visit her and to see some of that extraordinary country, including visits to Cairo and Luxor. Caroline was delighted to spend some precious time with her mother, and to see the life she had made for herself in Egypt, and of course Marylyn was overjoyed to have an opportunity to fuss over her expectant daughter. Me? I was just pleased to be amongst my loving new family; although my overriding memory of the trip is of the gruelling, incessant, inescapable heat. Although we had a great time, I think we were both relieved to come home to more manageable temperatures, especially Caroline who was by then three months pregnant.

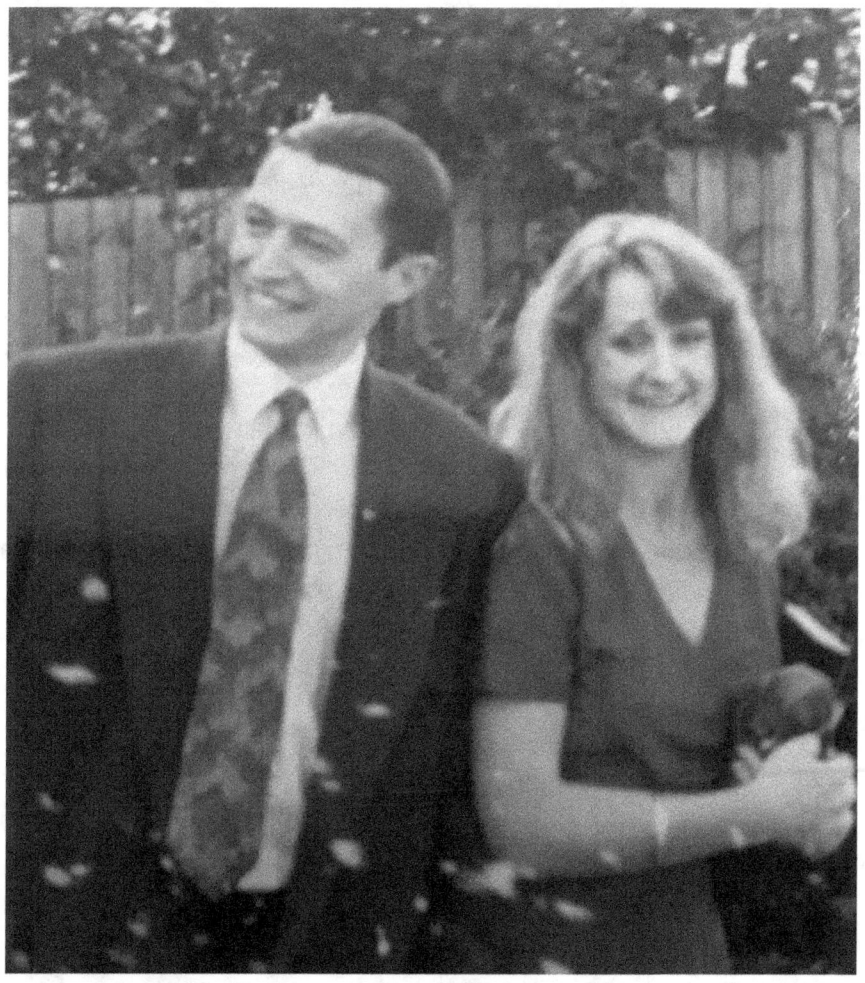

Caroline and me on our wedding day

Gran never got to see her great grandchild

Sadly, my grandmother died a few months before her great grandchild was born. Her death came as something of a surprise since there had been nothing to suggest she was close to death when I had visited her only a week earlier. She had of course grown frailer as she got older and had quite recently moved into a nursing home run by the Catholic nuns from our church. I had noticed on my last visit that she appeared less interested in things as I gave her my updates on Caroline's pregnancy and the latest news on our search for a new home. She maintained that she was very happy having gone to live with the nuns, and I was relieved that she would be well looked after in her new surroundings, with her beloved Sisters. But her time there was to be short; only a couple of weeks after my visit, I received a phone call from the convent advising me that she had passed away. When she was laid to rest, there were only a handful of mourners at the crematorium, close friends and family, and as I stood there listening to the priest's kind words, I thought back to my fears of all those years ago, after my mother had died, when I was terrified about what would happen to me if my grandparents died and I was left on my own. Now that day had arrived, far from the terror of being alone, I had a wife, good friends, a secure job, and would soon have a baby as well. I thought I would be alright after all.

Vernon made all the arrangements for her funeral and did a fantastic job which would have earned my grandmother's approval. It was a sad and sombre affair, and as with all these occasions the mourners' thoughts strayed to the memories of other departed loved ones. My grandmother's ashes were scattered close to the roses where my grandfather's ashes had been strewn. Some years later looking back on the day with my Uncle Vernon, he told me at the point of the scattering of the ashes, Keith had leaned over to him and said, "poor old Sonny, he's only had a few short years of peace, and now Agi is back with him, it will only be a matter of time before she starts her nagging again making his afterlife a misery as well". Although Keith had said this with a straight face in a suitably reverential tone of voice, Vernon said he had found it difficult not to laugh out loud at the image this presented.

Nana's legacy

For the next couple of months my mind was completely off my work. Fortunately, because I was largely responsible for managing my own timetable and daily workload, I was able to take a back seat for a while at work and find time to focus on the administration around settling my grandmother's small estate i.e., her flat. Even though she had lived a relatively modest life there were still funeral costs and what felt like exorbitant nursing costs from the last three months of her life spent at the convent nursing home (Sisters of Mercy? more like bandits in wimples!) to be sorted first. Nevertheless, I was able to sort everything and settle all Nana's matters appropriately, except for the minor matter of the proceeds from the sale of her flat. The proceeds were stated in her will as being due to come to me, a legacy of the fact that I had been named on the deeds of her house in Frimley Green, the money from the sale of which had been used subsequently to buy the flat she owned when she died. Unfortunately, my Uncle Richard had seen fit to contest the will, thereby adding considerable additional stress for me on top of having to deal with the rest of the probate and the preparation for the imminent arrival of my new baby. All the other Maure siblings were backing Richard in this formal claim, except for Vernon who came out in my support of my gran's desire to leave everything to me (no doubt he was very aware of his precarious position in this affair having nearly been responsible for their house being repossessed). After settling all the bills and proceeds of flat sale I was left with about £30,000. Not a vast sum by today's standards but I was just glad to bank the money and draw a line under the whole stressful affair. I could now move forward without being hassled daily on the phone by my disgruntled uncles and aunt.

Caroline had always got on well with my grandmother and enjoyed the stories she had told about the adventures from her life in Africa and her other life experiences. Most of all, Caroline was fascinated by my grandmother's tales of her clairvoyance, her sixth sense, and her dealings with the spirits of the after world. Caroline's fascination led to an amusing incident one evening during the latter stages of her pregnancy. On her way back from work, she had seen a sign outside a large house in Bromley advertising a psychic fair, and when she got home, she persuaded me to go along with her to take a look. We had never wanted to know the sex of our baby before it was born, but Caroline, by then only two weeks away from her due date, was desperate to hear what a fortune teller would say about the baby. So along we went and Caroline duly crossed the fortune teller's hand with silver (i.e. a £10 note) and followed her into a private room for the reading, during which a recording of the session was made for future reference (all part of the modern-day fortune telling service). Not wanting to distract the spirit medium's attention away from Caroline, I stayed outside, mulling about idly, vaguely aware of another female psychic talking to a group of people in the background. Suddenly this other psychic pointed at me and said, "you have the gift". She asked me if anyone in my family had psychic powers and somewhat embarrassedly, I mentioned my grandmother, to which the psychic replied a bit theatrically, in the manner of Madame Arcati, "there you are, you see but you don't see, you don't realise it, but you have the gift, if you choose to use it".

Just at that point Caroline came out of the room, and I took the opportunity of this distraction to exit with her and we went back to the car to listen to the tape of her session. In very broken English, the clairvoyant told Caroline that she would have a problem free, straightforward birth with the baby coming out easily - "whoosh", the old lady said as if to emphasise the ease and the speed of the birth that Caroline could look forward to. She further added that our child would be a healthy boy baby. Having listened to clairvoyants words again, this time together, Caroline and I hugged each other emotionally as we absorbed the implications of the glimpse into the future that we had just been given (our NHS antenatal scans and childbirth lessons were nothing compared with this). Two weeks later, following a very long, protracted, and difficult labour, which had lasted 36 hours, Caroline gave birth to our new baby, having in the end had to resort to a caesarean section instead of the natural birth she had hoped for. Not a "whoosh" in sight. Oh yes, and of course the predicted healthy baby boy turned out instead to be a beautiful and bonny baby girl. I hoped my grandmother had been a bit more accurate in fortune telling.

Fatherhood

Caroline gave birth to Joanne, a gorgeous and healthy, eight-pound baby girl, on the 22nd of March 1995. I cannot describe my emotions as the midwife passed Jo to me, to hold for the first time, other than to say it was the best experience I had ever had in my life, and I clutched the precious little pink snub nosed creature that I had helped create, close to my heart. After only about a week's paternity leave, I was quite pleased to get back to work and to resume a more normal pattern of life, going home at the end of each day to Caroline and Jo.

Caroline had opted to extend her maternity leave for an additional three months and so naively when Jo was just eight months old, we decided that the three of us should go on a weekend break to Berlin. On reflection we had obviously got a bit carried away with the romantic idea of us newlyweds enjoying these last moments of freedom with our new baby in such an historic and fascinating place as Berlin. Possibly at any other time of the year we might have got away with it, but we hadn't factored in the reality of coping with the freezing Berlin weather in December with a young infant. The trip turned out to be something of an nightmare; I was felled by food poisoning on the outward journey and was incapacitated for most of our first day in Berlin, then later Caroline and Jo came down with the same symptoms on our first evening. Although thankfully their illnesses were mild compared to mine, we were particularly concerned about Jo's welfare since we were aware of how dangerous prolonged vomiting and diarrhoea can be to a baby. To my relief however, mother and child's health quickly improved, and the break got better, so much so that by the following day we felt able to attempt the tourist spots. So, we left the hotel with Jo wrapped up warmly, insulated against the cold in her pram; the daytime temperature had dropped to about minus ten out on the streets! Jo fortunately remained as snug as a bug in a rug, and we managed to take in the sights. Despite our later separation and divorce, Caroline and I both retain very fond memories of that trip.

The black clouds start gathering

Caroline went back to work and a long working day, leaving

early and rarely getting home before 6pm. Because I had more flexibility in my timetable, one of my daily responsibilities became dropping Jo off at the childminder before work and then collecting her again on my way back home. I was trying hard to recover my mojo and to get myself back into the work ethic; but I was finding it increasingly difficult as I was constantly exhausted; no doubt due to a combination of stresses brought on from being a new father, interrupted sleep, and dealing with my grandmother's probate. Around the beginning of 1996, Caroline seemed to be going from strength to strength, she was fully back into her stride at work as an IT project manager for a firm of actuaries and was coping brilliantly in combining this with her role as the mother of a one-year-old. For my part, I was beginning to really struggle mentally again and found myself sinking back into distantly familiar feelings of hopelessness that I had hoped never to encounter again. I attempted to hide my true state of mind from Caroline, as I knew she had enough on her plate and because I believed I could work through it, like I had many times in the past. I don't think that I was experiencing full-on depression at that point, but I was finding it harder and harder to motivate myself to carry out what I needed to do to at least function normally in my job and at home. One evening after Jo had been put to bed knowing that I could no longer hide it from Caroline, I told her exactly how I was feeling. She was very understanding and supportive and encouraged me to make an appointment to visit our local GP surgery, which was only about half a mile from our house. I made an appointment and went to see my new GP, Dr P. Dr P was extremely sympathetic to my situation and listened attentively as I spoke about my current problems and gave her my lengthy case history.

When I had finished talking, Dr P shared some of her understanding of my condition together with some additional insights, which are worth reviewing here. She explained that it was not uncommon for the brains of adolescents who have been subject to a traumatic experience, such as the death of someone close to them, to trigger a strong chemical reaction which can result in tipping them into their depression (this was very much in line with the explanation of the possible cause behind my illness given to me by the consultant back in Frimley Park all those years previously). Additionally, Dr P theorized, that it was possible that I may have had a genetic pre-disposition towards becoming bipolar, that had been passed down to me from my mother; whose behaviours and mood swings suggest she was almost certainly bipolar. Whilst I wasn't and had never experienced some of the more extreme psychotic symptoms of the illness such as hearing voices, delusions of grandeur or other irrational beliefs like being able to fly, Dr P said that I had (and to some extent always would have) a very debilitating mental illness. And that the extreme mood swings I experienced in my youth were at least for now, being partially kept under control by my medication. She was confident that through continued adherence to my medication regime and being mindful at all times of my mood I could regain my normal lifestyle and get through life without any major problems. This all made great sense to me, and I took some comfort from her prognosis about the quality of life I could expect if I took care of myself. Under the circumstances Dr P went on to suggest to me a new drug that had relatively recently come on the market and had proven to be very effective in situations like mine. You've probably already guessed it, this new wonder drug that people were now popping to treat all sorts of depressive type disorders, was Fluoxetine (an SSRI "selective serotonin reuptake inhibitor) more commonly known to the likes of you and me by its brand name at the time "Prozac". On Dr P's recommendation I agreed to take the magic pills!

Hubble bubble, toil and trouble: the diagnosis

Having commenced taking Prozac, during my next couple of visits, Dr P stressed how important it was for me to get good sleep and where possible avoid thinking overly about my condition, to try and take each day as it comes, not to over worry and to avoid becoming over anxious. Sound advice but more difficult to put in practice. She advised that the effects of the Prozac would not be immediate but that after two or three weeks I should begin to feel as if a cloud was lifting and that my life should start to feel easier; it was just a matter of giving it enough time to let it kick in.

Over the next few months, I saw Dr P regularly as she wanted to monitor my behaviour, how I was feeling, and to check how my body was coping with any side effects of my medication. At that point she hadn't taken me off the Lithium completely but had instead reduced my "maintenance dose" from 1,200mg to 1,000mg per day. Any google search will quickly reveal that there are increased risks of combining the two drugs Lithium and Fluoxetine, from something called the "serotonin syndrome." These include a host of physical symptoms too long to mention here, but which at the more extreme end of the spectrum can include going into a coma and death - best avoided if at all possible, I think we can all agree. It was thought, and still is, that it is important to maintain a lithium level[9] in the bipolar patient to avoid the extremes of reckless behaviour which can be experienced from their mood swings. The safety check here being the regular monitoring of my wellbeing and my body chemistry.

After a couple of weeks of the changed medication regime, as

---

[9] Alternatives to lithium are often used in the case of bipolar patients who are intolerant or resistant to the effects of lithium.

Dr P had predicted, slowly but surely, I began to feel less tired, and a bit more positive and optimistic each day. So much so, that I no longer experienced the overwhelming mid-afternoon exhaustion that had become a characteristic part of my day; and I no longer felt the need to pull my car over to the side of the road for a mid-afternoon nap in order to be able to continue with my next set of broker visits. My mood did lighten and I stopped feeling as if I carried around the troubles of the world on my shoulders 24/7. I developed reserves of energy which meant that not only was I able to concentrate better at work, but at the end of the day I still had something left in my emotional fuel tank which allowed me to be more attentive and present for Caroline and Jo when I got home.

Socially I was back in business, able to enjoy myself a bit more, and I began waking up each morning feeling refreshed and more ready to face the day ahead. The crippling fatigue that is a common symptom of bipolar depression, was always one of the worst symptoms for me. I was constantly exhausted when I was in a downward cycle; and although I tried to battle through it for as long as I could, eventually it would become so complete and disabling that it robbed me of the ability to think or do even the simplest of things, at which point I would have to sleep, regardless of where I was. At work, things had started to improve; I was coping with my workload and organising my days more efficiently, I was beginning to function much more effectively, and crucially I was seeing the fruits of my labour in my results. In general, I was a lot more enthusiastic about everything I did, which in itself was a great tonic. I had managed somehow to maintain a reasonable level of physical fitness throughout and having recovered from a recurrent groin injury I regained my sharpness on the football pitch as well as in the workplace. Life was once again on an upward trajectory and in fact there were days when I was even beginning to enjoy myself once again.

As my mind cleared, I became engrossed in everything related to my work again and I re-acquired a lost interest of mine, namely stock market investments. In my younger days, as a lifelong "Red" I had participated in a very attractive bond offering that Manchester United had produced, which had given me a good financial return, and I had also dabbled in some of the privatisations of state-owned businesses like British Gas and British Telecom under the Thatcher government in the 1980s. Now I started investing again on a small scale and was pleased to make some money from these buys. At that time, a huge improvement in my enthusiasm and my motivation towards my work (I was now definitely on the up) combined with a burgeoning investment environment, meant that I was earning a lot more money than I had ever earned before. One disastrous consequence of what was fast on its way to becoming an all-consuming, almost obsessive focus on work and making money, which I didn't realise or appreciate at the time, was that I started devoting less and less physical or mental time or attention to those closest to me. This oversight would soon result in a loss to me which far outweighed any financial compensation I may have been gaining at the time.

It is hard to properly explain in words, but by the beginning of the Summer of 1996 I felt like my mind and my understanding of the world of finance was literally expanding exponentially around me. I was able to coolly navigate every negotiation challenge at work and I had finally become able to make confident, coherent, and compelling business presentations (a skill that had so eluded me in the past), all of which brought me more and more financial success. Like Bradley Cooper's character, Eddie Morra, in the film "Limitless" (although his enhanced cognition was as a result of the fictional nootropic drug NZT-48) it seemed that Prozac had given me a lift and had propelled me to higher levels of energy and confidence in everything that I turned my attention to. The effects of the Prozac combined with the lower levels of lithium I was now on (as a result of which I had shrugged off my feelings of exhaustion) left me buzzing with energy and ideas (uh oh- check bipolar mania alert); and far from needing to nap any more it seemed that there just weren't enough hours in the day for me to do what I needed to do, make money! Of course, my money making was all relative, I was no Gordon Gecko or Warren Buffet, but I was making a very good living at the time. Was I finally back on track and at a point where my boyhood potential, prior to my illness, suggested I should be? Or was this insanely productive and lucrative time in my life more attributable to entering a manic phase of my bipolar condition; which had been accentuated as a result of the change in my medication? Things were about to get even better... and then much worse.

Fully committed to this new way of being, I attended a further review meeting with Dr P, during which I explained to her that I was feeling much better and I was enjoying life again and looking forward to each new day. Perhaps I had been less than totally honest with Dr P about just how good I was feeling or how skewed towards work my life had become, because it came as a bit of a surprise when she suggested that perhaps it was time for me to stop taking the lithium altogether. She speculated that perhaps the trauma I had suffered from my mother's death, my teenage breakdowns, and the rest of my early life challenges had finally been resolved, and that now given my much more stable and balanced family man lifestyle (I can't possibly have been totally honest with her) I was no longer at risk from the extremes of my condition and therefore no longer needed to take the lithium. Perhaps over optimistically, and contrary to the hard lessons I had learned through the years of dealing with my condition, I agreed with Dr P's summary and recommendation, and I took the decision to try not taking the lithium; I left the surgery that morning feeling very pleased with her and myself as I ran down the street.

It turned out that this decision was to have disastrous consequences for me; now a quarter of a century on, it does seem rash that only a relatively few short months since my last depression, I came totally off the medication that had proven so critical in stabilising my mood swings over the last 15 years. The Journal of bipolar disorder seems to suggest that the use of anti-depressants alone is not effective in the long-term management of bipolar. Presumably though Dr P was following the recommended medical guidance available at the time (and of course the risks associated with long term lithium use were well known). I look back now and recognise this event for what it was; a failed experiment in coming off the lithium. However, the clarity, the levels of emotion, and energy fuelled optimism, loving and embracing life with conviction, inspiration, and passionate belief in everything I was doing was an experience I would not have missed. For a brief period instead of struggling though life I sailed; no, I sliced through it. It was worth taking a shot and I have absolutely no regrets about trying. In subsequent years, having gone back on lithium at a reduced rate, and still continuing to take Prozac, I have managed to maintain a more stable life from which I gain enjoyment, pleasure, and a wealth of emotional experiences (mainly positive). I am not sure that I am a better person, and sometimes feel thwarted in my aspirations but I have at least improved in understanding what matters in life including the interests of those people who are close to me.

As I write this, I can distantly remember the excitement and thrill that, at that time, I experienced from everything around me. My desire for understanding and knowledge was insatiable, but my labours remained tragically skewed in their goals, as I continued to put my energies far more into providing for my family financially than investing in the time I was spending with them. Perhaps this is my attempt at justifying the way I had become totally consumed by my job and all work-related matters, which no doubt I found more stimulating than the more emotional hard work and comparative boredom of home-life.

Critically for me, this period of renewed energy and creativity at work, coincided with Standard Life introducing a new charging structure for their products; which resulted in far greater transparency on the commissions being charged. For a variety of reasons this meant that the business relationship between myself and my brokers became a lot more symbiotic as we needed to work more closely towards maximising our mutual benefit from the contracts eventually issued. I quickly caught on to the opportunities that were available for us consultants working downstream from these changes, and I worked tirelessly at optimising the situation to my financial advantage, whilst at all times putting the interest of the clients first. All parties involved did a lot more business and at the time I used to smile at the thought of the words of the Hot Chocolate song, "everyone's a winner baby, that's the truth." This was certainly true as far as the insurance companies and the brokers were concerned although some years later after a lot of people lost a lot of money following bad advice about inappropriate pension transfers, the sector was forced to pay out around £11.8bn in compensation for mis-selling.

Because of my passion for investments of my own pension funds combined with some (albeit dated) knowledge of how the pensions sector works and fails at times, I would like to take a few moments to share my views on this scandal. A few years after I left the sector, the media brought to the public's attention, the scandal that had resulted following the introduction of personal pensions in the 1980s. Many people at the time received bad advice from pension experts, which resulted in them transferring existing pension benefits from employer schemes into private pensions. In a lot of cases not only did many people lose out on the guaranteed inflation linked, final salary benefits guaranteed to them under their old schemes; but their pension pots and retirement incomes automatically became subject to how well funds performed on the investment markets; in which there followed something of a crash. Of course, not all were losers, and for some the advice to transfer proved beneficial where they got out of poorly managed Employer schemes (who can forget the story of Robert Maxwell and the Mirror Group pension scheme fraud). Standard Life, like many other investment companies, emphasised the risks involved from leaving your earned pension pots with a previous employer's scheme, and we strongly recommended to people that they reviewed their situation with a broker or financial advisor. Many of these advisors were brokers whose incomes depended largely on them selling/transferring policies, which generated them commission every time they handled a pensions transfer, and as such they earned a lot of money in the process. Eventually many brokers around the country were struck off because of their involvement in this slightly dubious activity. At Standard Life, however, we took great care to make sure that in helping a broker to advise whether a client should or should not transfer out of a scheme we would provide a very comprehensive and transparent quotation, which enabled the individual pension holder to see a like for like comparison if they stayed in their existing scheme or transferred out and into a managed fund or a with profits fund into a new insurance company.

Okay, back to the plot. At the time, Standard Life employed about 425 consultants across the whole company (of which of course I was one). If I had been looking for any kind of objective measure, that would show just how effective I had become during this incredibly productive period in my life (which I attribute largely to my medication changes), there existed one; Standard Life had a league table that ranked its consultants by performance, and I was positioned virtually at the top, in the first half dozen names. When I think back to only half a decade earlier to memories of the video clip I had seen of the chaotic, insane, unintelligible presentation I had given in my attempt to become a consultant with Norwich Union, it was unbelievable that I was now one of the top performing consultants with a market leading company like Standard Life. Unfortunately, my time occupying these exalted heights was very brief and never to be repeated. And of course, in case I should delude myself too much it should be noted that this metric of my ability was limited in its scope and only reflected my professional performance; whereas by then I had already begun to seriously neglect other aspects of my life; in particular my marriage and my family, where I was about to become bottom of the league. For a while though, through sheer hard graft and determination I kept this up and was earning very good money, but inevitably at some point, I found that I wasn't able, or perhaps I wasn't willing, to keep all my plates spinning, and the crockery was beginning to smash big time in another part of my life.

Whilst the football season had ended, I was still keeping fit playing a lot of squash and five-a-side football. Both these activities involved a lot of contact with friends and as with my work life, my social life was also busy and hectic; I think I fooled myself at the time into thinking I was still achieving a good balance between family for love, and friends for socialising. I honestly don't remember exactly how it happened, but high on the misbelief that I was finally managing to live life to the full, I began to develop a different take on things (all real perspective had gone out the window), and my full on 90 mile an hour lifestyle demanded constant excitement and action. Set against this, the boring and mundane domestic life that I went home to each night was in stark contrast, and my feelings towards Caroline and our life together began to change. Caroline was still the same beautiful and wonderful young woman I had fallen in love with, but I couldn't resist the lure of the fast action life, with all its additional attractions, that awaited me just the other side of my front door. In essence my by now, distorted personality craved and insisted it was kept fed on a diet of the high life. Now that I had tasted what life could offer me, I couldn't help myself from reaching out and grabbing it. Indeed, I had already reached and taken some of what I wanted and thought I deserved already; and I liked what I had sampled. I became convinced that my desires could not be fully satisfied as long as I was required to go home to my role as husband and father each night and so impulsively and recklessly (see bipolar characteristics) I took the decision to leave Caroline and Jo behind and move out of our family home. I stayed a few nights at Paul's as he was about to go away, and I continued to party like it was going out of fashion, as well as continuing to work flat out. I felt great! As long as I managed to avoid thinking about Caroline and Jo, I felt no remorse, I simply followed my insatiable desire for action and adrenalin, like a junkie desperate to get high. This decision turned out to be a life changing, cataclysmic course of action for me, and one of which I was not really in control.

I have difficulty in remembering the precise details and sequence of events that happened next, I know I went back to Caroline and Jo for a short time, and then I moved out permanently and went to stay with a guy I knew, called Adrian, who had a house in Stockwell (close to the Swan although I think that was simply a coincidence). In my limited coherent thinking capacity at the time, I thought that at least work would be an easy commute for me from Stockwell. Almost on arriving at Adrian's however, it seemed as if someone switched off the light in my head. That first night as I lay in bed in that strange house, I instantly lost my confidence and my energy and drive as the enormity of my circumstances sank home. Just like when my mother had died, suddenly I felt completely alone again, in an unfamiliar house with someone I only vaguely knew and with the crushing knowledge that I had just thrown away everything I had ever wanted and strived so hard to achieve.

I was incredibly grateful to Adrian and his wife Sue, for putting me up like they did and providing me with a temporary roof over my head at my moment of crisis. The following morning, after getting almost no sleep, as I ritualistically drove myself to work I was on autopilot trying to compose and prepare myself for the day ahead and my mind was racing. In stark contrast to only a matter of days before when I had relished and harnessed this speed of light thinking to creative intent, now I couldn't even make sense of the traffic signs and road names that I drove past. Shaking and trembling, I pulled over and stopped the car and attempted to read some paperwork in advance of presentations I had to make later on that day, but as hard as I tried I simply could not process or comprehend the black and white shapes on the pages in my hands. The same feelings of anxiety and desperation from the night before washed over me, as I experienced a full-on panic attack and burst into uncontrollable tears (I'd been here before too). I tried unsuccessfully to get some kind of control of myself and think what to do. After a while, when the worst of the shaking had subsided, I turned the car around and to my shame did the only thing I could think of. I drove to Bromley and Caroline, my mental faculties in pieces and spiralling further and further away from the clarity I owed so much to, down into darkness.

Chapter 17 - What just happened?

Okay, time out! I have rushed at warp speed through the series of events, personally and professionally, that led up to the biggest crash and burn of my life, following the calamitous changes in my medication in early 1996. I know that on the face of it I don't come out well, and you would be forgiven for thinking it served me right and that I had brought all this upon myself; and that your sympathies are firmly with Caroline and Jo. But, as this story is fundamentally about my life in the context of my illness, I would like to pause and attempt to explain as best as I can, how I have subsequently made sense of how I came to be in the situation of the breakdown of my marriage (and my career as it turned out) only two short years after my wedding. At the time I was in no position to comprehend or understand what was going on for me, since I was too busy living in the eye of the storm. In the hyper-sensualised, euphoric state I was in during those few months, since having stopped taking the lithium, I had become totally consumed by one basic goal in life; to maximise my personal pleasure through experience. When writing it down now it seems pretty sordid and incredibly shallow, but at the time it was as if an all-consuming force, compelled me to act exclusively to satisfy my visceral needs; physical, mental, and emotional. I will admit my emotional needs were being driven exclusively by my libido, and what I sought in this department was simply sexual stimulation and satisfaction. I do not consider myself to be a bad person, or even a particularly selfish person (no more than the next man anyway,) but with the benefit of hindsight (what a lovely disclaimer for all our poor past decisions that single phrase gifts us) and a level of self-awareness I have since acquired, I recognise that I was at an acute level in my mental illness. All feelings for anyone around me, especially my loved ones, my wife and my baby daughter, i.e., people whose own needs conflicted with mine, were blocked out by the selfish ego trip I was pursuing pell-mell.

I firmly believe now that during this period, my chemically enhanced energy levels and mental activity had freed me of the dulling, anchor like effects of the lithium that had held me back for years. Worse still, added to this, I was then being propelled forwards by the rocket fuel of the Prozac I was taking. It was a recipe for disaster and the perfect storm that was about to hit. I wasn't able to make rational, informed decisions at the time, since I had passed beyond the reaches of objectivity. Instead, I was racing headlessly towards a precipice, on by far and away the biggest manic phase of my illness to date, one in which my behaviour was being driven only by base animal instincts, pursuing exclusively the satisfaction of my primeval desires at the cost of all else. I remember feeling a sense of righteous indignation and kidded myself that I was making up for all that I had missed out on for so long. In order to continue like that I had become conveniently blind to the collateral damage I left in my wake. Maybe at some level this self-justification was a form of self-protection created by my ID. It preserved my sense of entitlement to do what I wanted regardless of the costs, and it prevented me from total self-destruction under the weight of conflicted self-doubt. The result was similar to a modern-day Mr Hyde (although without the extreme excesses of that fictional character I hasten to add) I rampaged through the streets of South London, hell bent on sating my carnal desires.

At the beginning of this book, I listed impulsive behaviour, including a high appetite for risk taking, as being one of the common characteristics experienced by people during a bipolar manic phase. It has been well researched and written about that when someone with bipolar disorder is having a manic episode, reckless sexual behaviour and a significantly increased sex drive is quite common, in fact it can even be a warning sign of an impending manic episode This is not an attempt to excuse or justify my behaviour, "it wasn't me your honour it was the drugs that made me do it", and just in case I haven't made it clear, I take full responsibility and ownership for my actions. But my illness is an integral part of who I am, and at times it becomes the dominant factor in how I feel and behave. During this period, my illness, aided by the changes in my medication, does not make my behaviour acceptable by any standard, but hopefully it does make it a bit more explainable and understandable.

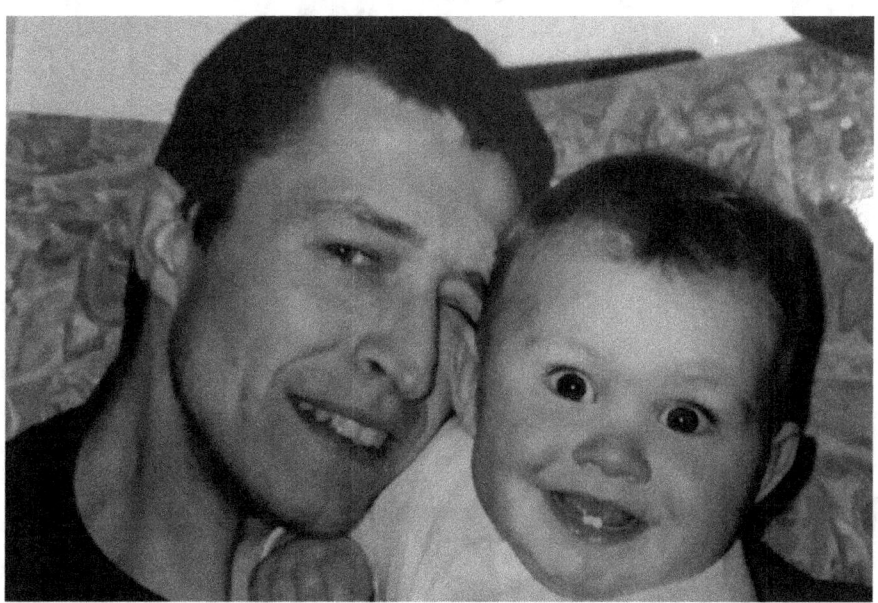

Above Jo and I when she was a baby and below more recently on one of my trips to the UK.

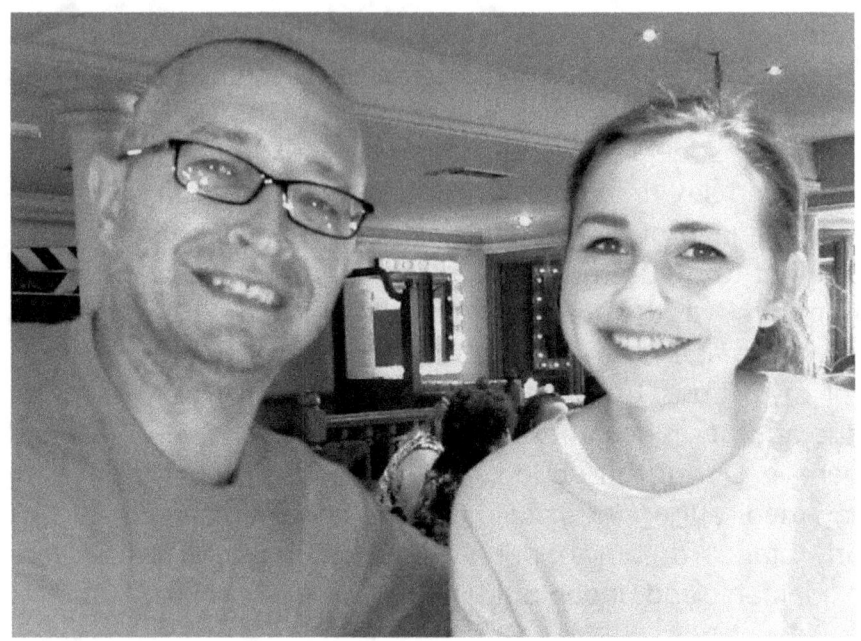

At the point at which I had moved out, Caroline and I had already stopped talking. My high-octane brain and frantic lifestyle had wholly taken possession of me and I had become completely uninterested in what I saw as the trivia of domestic/family life and in the irrelevance of small talk about mundane matters. Emotionally I had checked out of the marriage relationship and all commitments I had made to the shared responsibilities of running a home and jointly raising a child in a loving environment. But of course, this was the world that Caroline still occupied (on top of her day job) and although she attempted in vain to discuss household matters, towards the end I didn't even pretend to show any interest; this cruel behaviour on my part resulted in lots of arguments. I remember on one occasion, telling her "There are some things that I am just not that interested in, I have far more important things to think about, such as our financial future". This shows how I had ceased to be a participating member in our family life at the time. Caroline and I no longer slept with each other (you won't be surprised to know), I imagine my attitude and my alcohol enhanced snoring made me a very unappealing sleeping companion, and Caroline had banished me to the spare room. Despite all this, to Caroline's credit and my eternal shame, during this period, whilst I was behaving so appallingly towards her and Jo, she remained steadfast, tolerant and patient, perhaps hoping that I might turn back into the loving man she had married only a few short years before.

> **Caroline....**
>
> **We cannot change the past, and both our lives have moved on to a point where I believe we are happy and content, and hopefully able to see past the pain and look back on that crazy period for what it was. If you do ever read this, I hope that you will remember the good times as well as the bad. You took a chance on me (even when others had apparently cautioned you otherwise), my love for you was honest and heartfelt. You didn't deserve to be treated as you were, part of me will always love you and on some level, I know we were meant to be together at the time, if only to create our wondrous daughter, Jo.**

At that time, even by the standards of my previous manic episodes, I was behaving in an uncontrolled and bizarre fashion. I was only sleeping for three or four hours per night (just like Margaret Thatcher, makes you wonder doesn't it? - poor old Dennis). I was burning the candle at both ends as I devoted every waking hour to satisfying my pleasure receptors, spending too much time in bars and clubs with my friends; all the time in the back of my mind thinking, how can I get out of the boring domestic life I am tied to? Some dim distant part of my consciousness was saying that I shouldn't and couldn't and mustn't, but the chattering chimp in my head would not be kept quiet. I rationalised (ha!) that I had the perfect reason, "I am now a different person, things have changed, and my life has moved on". Such thoughts often came to me when I was swaying under the effects of alcohol in the Swan night club, drinking a beer, watching the young women dance tantalisingly on the dance floor, and getting high on the effects of the music that assaulted my senses and added to my feelings of dislocation. I told myself that I had to grab at this chance as it was the only way of achieving a more fulfilling and higher level of happiness. In order to achieve it, I had to leave my old life behind, I must focus on the gains not the losses. These and other similarly destructive thoughts slowly picked away stone by stone at the foundations I had built in my life, the cornerstones of my existence which had kept me safe and protected me from the mental demons of my early 20s. My thoughts were now taking over and leading me towards self-destruction and away from the stability I had so long sought (I wonder if Dr Jekyll experienced similar mental anguish? Perhaps it was Prozac he was necking from his conical flask!).

I have perhaps been a tad overly dramatic in describing what led me to my last (fingers crossed last) breakdown. The Jekyll and Hyde metaphor fits well though to explain how I have come to understand and make sense of what happened. Just as the honest God fearing, pillar of the community and scientific world Dr Jekyll, was changed into the monster Hyde by the well-intentioned potion he drank, so too I believe the changes in my medication meant that the worst aspects of my nature and my bipolar condition i.e., the manic me, came to the fore. I think it was as a direct result of the withdrawal of lithium, and the increase in my Prozac, that I lost control of any kind of self-regulation and the minute I was given the prescription changes my subsequent manic phase was all but guaranteed. Clearly since this change did not work out well for me, I went on to lose pretty much everything I held dear and which preserved me, and so you might expect me to speak bitterly, with anger, regret, and blame about these medication changes which led to my downfall, but to say such would be a lie. When reflecting whist writing this narrative, I have concluded that the clarity of thought I experienced at the time, the speed and precision with which I saw things in my professional life, the productivity and creativity I enjoyed, was like nothing I had ever experienced before or am likely to again. I cannot in all honesty say that I regret this brief chance to live to my full potential; maybe this was what I had missed out on. But predictably, like a bulb that burns brightest just before it expires, it was not sustainable (I imagine many an ex-heroin or cocaine addict might speak similarly) and predictably, inevitably, like a moth drawn towards a flame, once more I crashed and burned.

Chapter 18 - Monday morning blues

Okay, time out over; I'm back at the wheel of my car on the Monday morning after my sleepless night at Adrian and Sue's, unable to get my shit together sufficiently to even consider going to work, and like a homing pigeon, the only thing I could think to do was to set a course for home and pray that Caroline would take pity on me enough to provide me with a temporary refuge. At the time, if I imagined that I couldn't sink any lower than I already had, that I was at rock bottom, I was sorely mistaken, as I had still much further to fall. Over the next few weeks my mental state deteriorated still more to the point that I was almost unable to string two words together or to piece together any coherent thoughts. I was in tatters and on top of being an emotional wreck I was simply unable to do anything but sleep and smoke and watch TV in a semi-comatose state. There was no doubt that I was having another mental breakdown and deep in the recesses of my consciousness I was able to associate this with my medication changes. Together with Caroline's help, I manged to make an appointment to see Dr P. Upon seeing me she immediately recognised the perilous mental state I was in, and also concluded that coming off the lithium had been the catalyst. Dr P wrote me out a prescription there and then, re-instituting my lithium regime, and I mentally resigned myself to the fact that lithium and I were going to be companions for the rest of my life. I had always been aware that there were potential harmful side effects from the long-term use of lithium e.g., the mental deadness and the liver damage, which is why I had welcomed the opportunity to come of the drug in the first place, but enough was enough, time to wake up and smell the coffee.

Initially, Caroline was supportive and understanding of my illness and my situation and she showed great tolerance of how I was around the house, unable to start or complete even the simplest of tasks. Unspokenly, we knew our marriage and any future together was of course over. Whilst my illness put some context and explanation around my behaviour leading up to me leaving home, there was no coming back from what I had done and how I had treated Caroline and Jo. I was under no illusions that my presence there was being tolerated only because I was unwell, and even then, only until I got sufficiently well enough to move on/out. With time, I started to feel a little better, but I was still having real trouble with communicating. My close friends Keith and Paul were shocked at the state I was in, they could see how I was struggling (my near total silence and tearfulness were a dead giveaway) and were secretly wondering if this was a permanent vegetative state I had moved into.

During this period, I recall visiting Keith's dad Les in Salisbury, which was a nice get away for me, providing some temporary relief from the reality I was living. Whilst I don't have much memory of the visit it was just good to be with people that cared about me, including Keith's sister and brother-in-law who lived very close by. This was familiar territory to my recoveries back in my late teens. Ordinarily, amongst their company we would have been laughing and re-telling old tales and taking the mickey out of one another, but on this occasion, I was a shell of the person they knew and although I was there physically, I was to all extent and purposes a silent guest as my brain was in lockdown and had disconnected all communication channels. However, simply to be with familiar, friendly faces was comforting to me, although I don't suppose they realised just how much this meant. People who know me would vouch for the fact that in normal times, I am relatively engaging in social situations and describe me as articulate (or at least vocal) and always ready to voice an, often contrary, opinion on a range of subjects (prior knowledge or consideration of the subject matter was never a limiting factor for me), but at that time I was an empty vessel. Like a zombie or Randle McMurphy post lobotomy, in One Flew Over the Cuckoo's nest, the lights were on but there was no one at home. I was beyond caring how I was perceived by others, by most definitions I was not a functioning human being.

Unsurprisingly I had been immediately signed off work on sickness leave, and although my employer was extremely sympathetic to my situation, the longer I was off the more questions started to be asked by human resources on the exact nature of my illness. As my sick notes were repeated and I was in my second month of sick leave I was aware that my firm was now more closely monitoring my situation. Of course, this was normal procedure for any employer interested in the recovery and well-being of a member of their workforce, but for me it was one more concern on top of everything else. In the meantime, there was some change at home; I was less obviously anxious and whilst I still shunned any interaction with anyone outside of the family (how the tables had turned), Caroline decided that a break would be good for my recovery, so the three of us went to Lanzarote for a week. Although there had been some easing off in my crushing depression, I remained incapable of any kind of straight thinking, I still had major self-confidence issues and my communication abilities remained in the pan, but the fact that I was able to even contemplate making this trip hinted at a sign of recovery.

After a couple of months, the lithium was definitely doing its thing again, as evidenced by the fact that my thought processes were stabilising, and my general cognition had improved.

Although far from 100% I was feeling a lot better, sufficiently well enough to contemplate my situation, to dip a toe tentatively back into the real world I had so spectacularly bailed out of a few months earlier. Naturally, my job was at the top of the list. Fortunately, prior to my breakdown I had been riding high at work, after all I had a chemically enhanced track record that demonstrated my value to the company, and my reputation was hitherto untarnished. On my return everyone in the office showed me nothing but kindness and concern and expressed sincere messages of support. Several people commented that after all, what had happened to me could have happened to any of them (I was very content for them to reach that conclusion even though I was doubtful of the truth of it). They all went out of their way to welcome me back and make me feel at ease. Tea, sympathy, and understanding amongst my office colleagues was one thing, but it was clear to my managers and abundantly obvious to my brokers that I could not be relied upon to provide them with the information and support they needed to do the Standard Life business they wanted to. In short, the commonly held view (and one that I secretly shared) was that I was not up to doing my old job, and like a vicious circle that increased my stress levels at every rotation, I soon began to feel more useless, worthless, and hopeless than ever, so much so that only a month after my return to work, I went off sick again.

Throughout this whole episode of illness and recovery, I never once felt like taking my own life. I think I still harboured deep feelings of resentment towards my mother for killing herself and abandoning me. Having said that, there were many nights when having retired to the sanctuary of my bed, I entertained thoughts that it would be great not to wake the next day and just to be free from the hell I was living in. What a stark contrast to the electric emotions of just a few months earlier when I was only sleeping four hours a night and rueing the fact that there were only 24 hours in a day.

Once again, with my tail between my legs I returned to see Dr P for another sick note. I took some small encouragement from the fact that I was now in a slightly improved state and better able to communicate to her what was happening and how I was feeling (improved at least in comparison to the train wreckage state I had been in when I last saw her). After some discussion we agreed that the best course of action would be for me to continue with what I had come to view as my life saver, my precious lithium, but instead of the 1,200mg a day I had been on my dosage would be reduced to 1,000mg. It was also decided that I should continue with the Prozac at a 20mg dose whilst we attempted to find the right balance of the two drugs for me. Progress was painfully slow and was much longer than everyone (Dr P, Caroline, and me) expected. So, I sat at home in a funk, doing next to nothing to help myself, smoking heavily (I had by then developed a full-on nicotine addiction) to pass the time, no longer concerned over my lifetime obsession with keeping physically fit. As the months passed, despite myself, I did find that I was feeling a little better about things and importantly a bit more optimistic, and eventually I felt ready to try another return to work, after all I couldn't stay like this for ever – could I?

This time, a very different welcome awaited me from my managers. It was apparent that they had been talking and planning for my eventual return. On my first day back, I was led into my boss's room where it was explained, pleasantly but firmly, that after talking with Head Office it had been agreed that I could no longer look after my panel of brokers. This news was devastating to me after all the hard work I had spent to gain the trust and understanding of my brokers, the results of which had been good for everyone, as evidenced by the mutual financial success we had all enjoyed. I had begun to think of many of them as my friends and we had socialised regularly; maybe a friendship that had been in part buoyed by my entertainment expense account, which I had wielded as a tool of my trade. Instead, my boss went on to offer me a more junior consultants' role, which was effectively a demotion since I would once again be a development consultant, working with a bunch of quasi brokers who did little in the way of pensions and investment business (this would be similar to the bad old days at Prolific). Of course, even if I could prove myself up to this new position, something I had grave doubts about, such a move would have meant a massive drop in my earnings due to the lack of any commission whist I developed my new patch. I understood instantly what was happening, I was now judged a high risk and if I insisted on staying with the company, they intended to side-line me into an unimportant role where I could do no damage. So, it was no surprise when an alternative offer was also put on the table. I could leave under a redundancy agreement, with a modest financial settlement, and retain my pension entitlement intact. Just to add to this, they played some hardball by pointing out to me that I had not been completely honest (i.e., you lied to us) when I joined them, by failing to disclose my ongoing treatment for my bipolar condition. I was told to take a few days to decide and let them know my decision.

I spoke with one of my brokers, Pat, who had become a good friend and he put me in contact with a lawyer friend of his, who agreed to help me consider and better understand the options, their implications, and their relative merits. As I discussed it with the lawyer, it quickly became a no brainer really; I couldn't face going back into the office to work, I didn't think I could cope with developing the new patch of brokers, and I couldn't survive financially without the commissions I had come to rely on. Whilst the decision was inevitable, it was nonetheless an incredibly sad day for me. I had fought so hard and come so far (from the inept administrator at Crown Life, to the babbling idiot giving the panel presentation to become a consultant at Norwich Union to eventually achieve my goal of being a high performing pensions consultant at Standard Life). I had continued to roll the dice at every step, but finally I had to concede that the game was over. I agreed to the redundancy offer there and then, and left the office that day never to return.

I returned to doing what I had become best at, sitting around the house, staring at the same four walls, and feeling sorry for myself. I occasionally met up with a few friends just to see people apart from Caroline and Jo, and as a break from the monotony. In particular, I spent quite a bit of time with Paul, staying over regularly at his house and going out for the occasional beer, at times able to briefly forget about my sorry circumstances. Meanwhile at home, my continued lethargy and inactivity was beginning to take its toll on Caroline's nerves. I guess I wasn't the only one who was having to put their life on hold. Caroline had patiently tolerated this situation for over six months and no doubt wanted to move on as well, and it was certain that any plans she had for achieving future happiness did not include me. Eventually, her patience worn thin and exasperated by any obvious lack of effort on my part to improve my situation, she insisted I once again go back to the doctors. This time, Dr P tentatively suggested that I go for a week's assessment in the psychiatric ward at our local hospital (isn't this where we came in?) I do wonder if this suggestion was as much about giving me a change of setting and getting me out of the house for a short while, so as to give Caroline some respite. Whilst having a mental illness can be a terrible thing and can be debilitating for the sufferer to live with, so can living with someone with a mental illness be incredibly challenging and exhausting. In Caroline's case, day in and day out she was living with my black shadow in the house sucking any joy or positive emotions out of the atmosphere and seemingly exerting no effort or urgency to change. Not a positive place to live in or bring up a young child. Added to this, the elephant in the room, our marriage which was effectively over, meant that for Caroline to move on, I had to move out. I understand the strains that this must have put her under and I am once again truly grateful that she didn't just kick me out onto the street.[10]

Another bad start to the year – 1996

Having completed a period of rest and recuperation (it sounds more acceptable when described like this) of about six days in the psychiatric unit of the Kent hospital, and after a further week or so back in my daily pattern of lying around the house, Christmas arrived which provided a temporary distraction from my misery as I made an extra effort to transfer my attentions away from my own misery and onto Jo who was about to experience her second ever Christmas.

I had by then come to the opinion that there was no future for me in which I was a somebody again, and I believed that at the ripe old age of thirty-three, my life was over, and my fate lay forever within the four walls of my house, as I had no desire to ever venture outside again (I am sure Caroline had a different take on things). I cannot remember the exact catalyst for the subsequent change, and it may be purely coincidental, but, having resigned myself to this awful future, I began to relax and even started to regain some lost energy. My brain began to

---

[10] A multinational piece of research published in 2011 in the Acta Psychiatrica, Scandinavia, found that mental illness increased the likelihood of divorce by up to 80%, and there is a vast amount of research and literature covering the challenges on maintaining relationships where one of the partners suffers with bipolar.

work semi-properly again, partly perhaps because I was sleeping better and more restfully at night- the consequence of this was a gradual but steady rehabilitation of my frazzled mind. By the time of my 33rd birthday at the end of January 1996 the black cloud that had shut out all light in my life since my latest breakdown had begun to lift. Finally, there began to slowly emerge some daylight and colour, tone and nuance in my life. I understand now that my bipolar condition is one in which I moved between extreme highs and crippling lows. Medication could help with the extremes, but my illness would take its own pre-determined path despite external interventions. My own behaviour and the cavalier changes in my medication had precipitated my latest boom and bust, and only rest and the passing of time had pulled me through. But it had not been without cost, at the end of this latest swing of the pendulum, I had lost my marriage, my job, my prospects, and any sense of who I was. At least now my mojo and my lithium levels had returned sufficiently for me to consider the future more optimistically, and crucially I knew that I had some influence in the making of it. I now felt that I had enough energy to get off my arse, take some control, get busy, and earn some money.

Chapter 19 – The Phoenix rises

As I emerged from my depression I had tentatively begun driving again. I found the challenge of having to concentrate exclusively on this complex task, helped focus my mind, and that it was also strangely mentally stimulating. Who knows, maybe the intellectual processing power required to negotiate my way safely through the streets of London, without harming myself or any innocent bystanders, reactivated some dormant neural pathways in my brain that had taken a six-month sabbatical. Anyway, whilst driving to Paul's one day I was passing through Stockwell, and I was reminded of the army of minicabs that were always waiting outside the Swan late at night, eager to give punters a ride home in exchange for, what felt like at the time, large amounts of cash. This thought stayed with me while I sat around at Paul's and it continued to percolate in my head (there wasn't a huge amount else going on in there at the time). On a whim I decided to check out what was required to become a mini cab driver; how hard could it be I reasoned? After all I had access to a car, not mine I know, but that was a minor detail, and I had a lot of experience of driving in South London from when I went to meet with my brokers, so I was confident that I could find my way from A to B (I probably should have given that last assumption a bit more probing). It transpired that these attributes, together with my clean driving licence, made me more than qualified for the job, and the dodgy cab firm I contacted, welcomed me with open arms, explaining that they were always looking for new competent drivers. It was all so easy; I was immediately issued with a radio/walkie talkie and we agreed that I should start the following evening when demand was at its peak (not for me any gentle easing in). The next day I invested in a new road atlas of London and with the addition of a large street map of South London (for surely, they wouldn't send me north of the river) spread out beside me on the passenger seat I set off. In my mind if anything, I was over prepared.

No sooner had I turned it on, the radio began chattering with instructions from the office providing the essential information for my next pick up. It probably won't come as any surprise to any of you that have managed to stay with my story this far, to learn that I struggled from the outset, immediately realising that I had wildly over-estimated my street knowledge of South London. On being given the details of a job from the controller, I first had to locate the destination of the pick up on the map, then invariably I had to work out where the fuck I currently was. Next, I had to somehow plot a route between the two points and finally I had to submit my immediate next turns to memory. For me, it was going to be less a case of getting from A to B, and more a case of having to break each journey down into A +1 and A +2 if I was ever going to get to B (where was Google Maps when I needed it?) It was around then, that reality kicked in and I remembered how difficult I had found traveling to my brokers' offices initially. I was always late, never on time, and often when lost I would have to re-trace my steps back to where I started in order to try again. Whilst the newly emerging, positive me said, "stick with it, you will pick up on the techniques and tricks of finding your way round", no matter how hard I tried I continued to get hopelessly lost, despite my best efforts. Over the next few days, I was lost more often than not, and I constantly rebuked myself along the lines of "just find out where you are first and then we can worry about where you have to get to after that; simple!" The few fares I did get barely covered the cost of my fuel and the only real gain I made was in losing a few pounds of weight through nervous sweating whilst driving around in circles. Looking back on it now, I can laugh. It must have been immediately apparent to my passengers that I was a clueless rookie, not least because as soon as they were settled in their seats, I introduced myself, and told them that I fully intended to get them to their destination safely and on time, but that in order to do so they would have to give me directions.

On my third and final day (yes, I lasted three whole days), I was given a job to pick up a small child from a school, somewhere in London and deliver him to his home, at some other place in London (what were they thinking of giving me such responsibility). Finally arriving at the school pickup, about twenty minutes late, I hurried the child into my car, which was by that stage full of a fog of my cigarette smoke (in just three days of taxi driving my cigarette consumption had developed to near chain-smoking proportions), explaining to him that due to an unforeseen delay we needed to make up for lost time. It was this last traumatic journey that put the final nail in the coffin of my taxi driving career and convinced me I was in the wrong line of work. The small boy, who only minutes earlier had appeared so happy and care free, sat back and nervously fastened his seat belt, no doubt assuming that his role in his journey home, would as normal, be that of a passive passenger. I've got news for you bucko! I thought as I reached back and handed him the A-Z. Alas, it turned out that the young man, aged about eleven or twelve, had never paid any particular attention to his route on his previous journeys and was clueless as far as following map directions were concerned (why on earth don't they teach reading an A-Z as a basic life skill at school). So, before we could even set off, I had to spend an additional 20 minutes educating him on the basics of map reading (I had only been allocated 45 minutes for the whole gig). I looked earnestly into his eyes, which were by now streaming with tears from all the cigarette smoke, and told him that it was going to take team work to get him home, and if he ever wanted to see his mother and father again, we needed to work together. Fortunately, I think he found the whole thing a bit of an adventure, or a life lesson even, as he certainly got to see parts of his neighbourhood that he had never seen before. On arrival at his home, considerably later than anticipated, his parents rushed towards the car, they appeared just as relieved to see him arrive as I was to see him go.

I had thought my job at Standard Life stressful, but it was as nothing compared to mini cabbing. Added to my total incompetence in knowing where I was going, traffic jams, road works, and detours provided further additional variables to overcome - as if I needed more challenges! At least now with my mental faculties restored, it was crystal clear to me that I would never make a good taxi driver and so having left the kid with his tearful parents, I headed back to the taxi office and returned their radio and equipment as well as their share of my fares. I probably cleared about twelve quid in my entire three-day career as a cab driver, but in truth I think I got away lightly. I shudder to think of the number of near collisions I had on the road when trying to read a map and drive at the same time. On a positive note, I had come through this adventure mentally unscathed (not sure I can say the same for my passengers), I still had a clean driving licence and it felt great to have dipped my toe back into society. Added to this my sense of humour was returning as I smiled to myself at the thought of the new tales I had added to my repertoire.

Over the next few weeks my focus in life shifted away from my internal wretchedness and onto the world outside of my head and home, as I started paying more attention to what was going on in the wider world. I was furiously thinking about what on earth I was going to do in the short term for a job and in the longer term for some kind of career. I remembered how my old friend, Paul Simpson, had left his boring work as a pension administrator and gone on an adventure to the Czech Republic to teach English. I thought on this some more; in principle there was nothing to stop me doing something similar, Caroline I was certain, would be relieved to see me go. Just as with the cab driving, I started considering the entry requirements for such a career change, I knew that it would take more than just a car and a clean driving licence. From talking to Paul, I knew that the minimum requirement to teach English abroad was to hold the Teaching English as a Foreign Language Certificate (TEFL). I remembered Paul working intensively and attending classes three nights a week over a 13-week course to gain this gateway qualification; further research showed me that the course wasn't cheap, coming in at around £750. Eventually I concluded that I may no longer have had a car, but I did have a working command of the English language, okay it wasn't my strongest suit, but surely, I would be at least one step ahead of a Czech student coming totally new to the subject. The more I thought about this possibility and how it had provided Paul with a chance to reinvent himself with a totally new life in a new country, the more convinced I was that I should give it a go. Also, I recalled from my one previous trip to Prague back in 1989, that a round of six beers cost only a quid, so perhaps there were other advantages to be had as well. The money may not be great, but the cost of living was significantly cheaper than in the UK and Paul had said that an English teacher could live a comfortable existence in the Czech Republic. After my recent experiences, happiness rather than financial success, was what I was aiming for and I desperately needed a purpose and a focus to take me through the next phase of my life, which would include decoupling from my wife and daughter.

I went through a kind of mental checklist, ticking off the different boxes; I had plenty of spare time, some leftover cash from my redundancy, and crucially a total absence of any better ideas, so I signed up to take the TEFL course. I told myself that even if I didn't ever go on to teach abroad, it would be useful to have the qualification, and I kept coming back to how happy Paul had seemed in his new life in a new country, compared to how miserable and despondent he had been when working in London in the pensions industry. In the end I didn't take the thirteen-week part-time course option, preferring instead a full time, four-week intensive, Monday to Friday course, for the same price; at the end of which there would be an examination and if I passed, my certification to a new life.

Initially I found the course incredibly difficult, and I wondered if perhaps the 13-week course would have been a better option for me, providing me with more time to assimilate my learning and to do some additional background study. Not only did the course cover the structure and grammar of the English Language, it also included teaching skills, the pedagogy of learning, and developing and adapting materials for use in lessons. Just as with my mini cabbing experience, I quickly learned that I had massively overestimated my existing subject knowledge, in this case, the English Language. I wouldn't have known a gerund or a modal verb if they had bitten me on the arse, and making myself clearly and succinctly understood by others was, as we have seen, something I had struggled with even when I was an expert in the subject matter. I think knowing that this was the only show in town for me helped, and also knowing that I had through persistence eventually overcome my inability to give group presentations (hold on though, was that me or was it the meds?) helped; either way I worked desperately hard and just about managed to keep up with the course demands. I was the oldest student on the course by far, the majority of the other students were university graduates, seeking out an alternative, more interesting and diverse career to that of teaching in the UK. The graduate students discussed amongst themselves how hard they were having to work compared to when on their degree courses. Meanwhile I tentatively congratulated myself that, as someone who had dropped out of two degrees, it looked like I was finally going to complete a course that I started. Gradually I was beginning to feel more confident about my choice, I was becoming more familiar with the grammar, I was picking up tips on effective teaching, and I was writing lesson plans. I was even teaching the odd practice lesson to foreign students on study visits to London. I was incredibly busy, but I was coping and beginning to believe in myself again.

Towards the end of the third week, we received a visit from the owner of a language school in Poland who was looking to sign up recruits to teach at his school. I listened to what he had to say about his school, about the jobs on offer, about his city Kielce, and about Poland more generally. It sounded similar to how Paul Simpson had described his experience of the Czech Republic. Crucially, both were former soviet bloc countries with emerging opportunities, cheap beer, cheap fags, and a great lifestyle for an exotic teacher of English from London, such as me. I persuaded Richard, a student colleague I had become friendly with, to enrol as well. Richard was 23 and he held a degree in history and religion; he definitely did not intend going into the priesthood and would sooner shoot himself than take up a teaching post in a school in England. I liked Richard a lot, he was the first new friend I had made in a long time, he was enthusiastic, optimistic and looking for adventure in the wider world as he moved towards the maturity of his mid-twenties. I am not sure I was his best choice as mentor for this, but it was too late, I had already rolled the dice.

A week later, the final assignment of the course was to teach a full lesson to a group of selected foreign students. As well as teaching some grammar, we were required to present something which the students could discuss. I chose a recording of "A Boy Named Sue," by the late, great Johnny Cash, and asked the students to discuss what the message was behind the song lyrics. Although my lesson was not the best lesson the students received that day, and I didn't qualify top (or anywhere near top) of the class, my presentation was deemed good enough to get me through. I had enjoyed the course, and it had done my self-esteem the power of good to successfully complete it. On finishing and being awarded our TEFL qualifications, Richard and I were given dates by Marick Paneck, the owner of the language school in Kielce, for when we would begin our new life as teachers in Poland.

The last few weeks in England

Finally, I again had a future and something to look forward to. Yes, this future was tinged with sadness as it would signify the end of my marriage and mean that I would be leaving Joanne behind, but my overriding emotions were of relief, excitement, and optimism. I had somehow weathered another bipolar storm, as evidenced by the fact that I was I was still here, and that which does not kill me makes me stronger (according to Nietzsche at least). I was fairly certain that the medication change had been the cause of my last episode, and I was determined never to tinker with my lithium again (although that wasn't the first time I had vowed that). Then just like back in the summer of 1981, after I had successfully completed my A-Levels and awaited the next chapter of my life to start, I had a few weeks to kick back, before I travelled to Poland. I felt I could really let my hair down, relax, and enjoy the time. Caroline and I, having discussed my plans, both acknowledged that our short marriage had come to an end and that my move to Poland appeared a good one as my options in England were limited. She wished me well and generously offered that I could stay at the house whenever I returned to the UK on visits to keep up my contact with Jo. By this time, I had signed over the house to Caroline and we had settled on an amount of maintenance that I would pay towards Jo.

Over the next few weeks, I took great pleasure in rekindling my social life; meeting up with old friends who I hadn't seen much of during my illness. Once again, I took to the nightclub scene with Paul Nolan and Tony Werner and Steve Kenny; Steve was back doing some business in London. It felt a little strange to hear myself chatting to women in the clubs, explaining that I was a qualified English teacher, and would soon be heading off to Poland. They weren't to know it was a lightweight bullshit qualification; and after having repeated it a few times to different women (I was back playing the numbers game) I began to think myself into my new life. When I look back, I remember this period as being a wonderful little interlude, which marked a transition for me into my new life. I was back in control, back in the saddle, and I even managed a few tentative jumps along the way (boom boom). On one of my last nights in the UK, I went to a Club in the City with Paul and Tony, where I met and danced with a very attractive forty-two-year-old Danish woman. She was in London for a brief vacation and at the end of the night I went back with her to her hotel. It turned out that she was returning to Copenhagen the next day and in the spirit of adventure, I suggested that I could perhaps deviate my journey to Poland via Copenhagen, stopping off to visit her on the way. This was probably a ridiculous decision as it certainly used up some of my precious diminishing reserves, perhaps my brain still wasn't firing on all cylinders. Flying to Copenhagen and then taking the train to Poland was more than a little extravagant and expensive, but at the time it felt like a sexual adventure and my western European swansong. Which is exactly what it proved to be. The woman had a fantastic apartment, she took me on a tour of Copenhagen, we visited a few bars, and we went to a World War II historic site where the Nazi's had made plans for the Final Solution (nice!). After only a couple of nights the woman told me it was time for me to leave, I noticed she had some photos of a small girl in the flat, who I took to be her daughter, and this was fine by me. Although I felt a little bit as if I had been dismissed as my usefulness was over (what did I say about night club romances?), this was though, in fact fine by me. She generously dropped me off at the train station and my travel arrangements to Poland continued.

Chapter 20 - Polska here I come

At the age of thirty-four I was now embarking on a journey to a brand-new life; one which I hoped would be full of Eastern, or at least Eastern European, promise. As I sat in the train compartment watching the rolling fields whizz past, I told myself that I was running towards a new life not running away from my old one (a small but important distinction for my self-esteem). I was not so much giving up on a way of life, but instead like so many economic migrants before me, I was heading towards what I trusted would be a new and different life, laden with new opportunities and chances. It was true that this was not the life I had envisaged for myself when I had been riding high only a year earlier in London, but this was the way the dice had rolled - "It is what it is", so they say. I did not hold my illness or my medication blunders, wholly responsible for my actions, for after all where did my condition end and where did I start? Surely my illness, quite probably passed onto me in my genes from my mother, was as much a part of me as my blue eyes or my curly hair. I was not defined by my condition but at critical times in my life, my condition had exerted such an influence on my behaviour, as to result in life changing events for me. As Poland drew ever closer, I didn't know if or for how long I was going to be okay for, but I did know one thing, that I was going to make the most of every minute I could towards building my new life.

On March 30, 1997, I arrived in Kielce where I was met at the train station by my new boss Mareck Paneck. Mareck thoughtfully had picked me up to ease my introduction into this strange new city and to take me to the flat he had arranged for Richard and myself to live in. The flat had two bedrooms and was on the seventh floor of a fairly modern (by Polish standards anyway) apartment block. After a quick meal and a few beers with the two other housemates we were to share with, Richard and I decided to explore our new neighbourhood a little; we were excited and animated having finally arrived in our new lives, and we were eager to get an early taste of the adventure we had come to this strange land in search of. This probably wasn't the most sensible preparation for our first real teaching which was timetabled for the following day, nor was the fact that in our enthusiasm to get out there neither of us took any notice of our surroundings or where we wandered, although Richard had thought to bring with us a note on which he had written our new address. Kielce was actually a city; in fact, it is the fifth largest city in Poland (by population) and we had no knowledge of the layout of the city and no ability to read anything in this new foreign language.

We soon found ourselves in a bar where we met a Polish/American guy called Mareck and his Polish girlfriend Mariola. Not long after, two female friends of theirs turned up, Kasha and Monika. I was immediately attracted to Kasha, who I felt had a streak of wildness about her, and Richard, happily for both of us, struck up a conversation with Monika. We were in heaven, our first night in Poland and we were making friends with the locals (thank God they could speak a little English). When it got late, being responsible English teachers with a busy day teaching the following day, we made arrangements to meet the two girls again and we left setting off into the streets of Kielce again. But now in the dark, things looked very different and unfamiliar, and to make matters worse Richard had lost the piece of paper with our address written on it. In vain we wandered around the streets for about half an hour, seeking anywhere that looked familiar. Finally realising that this was not going to happen, we were both freezing by then (oh, did I not mention it had started to snow?), in desperation we booked ourselves into a hotel near the station. It was beginning to feel like this probably wasn't the best preparation for our first day teaching. To top it all off I was wearing contact lenses, and without any means of storing them in a sterilised way overnight, I decided to sleep with them in. And so it was that the following day, having had very little sleep, done zero preparation, and almost blind by virtue of the irritation and mist that had formed in my eyes from my contact lenses, Richard and I turned up at the language school to teach. I wish I could say we learned a lesson from this experience, but that would be a lie; preparation and planning was never my strong suit.

And now, over two decades on, here I am still in Poland (my home now), living in the historic University City of Wroclaw, in the Southwest of the Country. I am happily married and live with my wonderful Polish wife, my two teenage Polish sons, and our four dogs. We live in a comfortable house on the outskirts of the city and what's more, I own two flats in the centre of Wroclaw, which I rent out to university students to supplement my income. This last point is a good job too as my earnings from my English teaching have just about dried up, although my main work these days is in actively managing my modest stocks and shares portfolio. I am still in regular contact with my daughter Jo in England, who is now all grown up and doing very well for herself also in the world of investments and finance. She visited me again recently with her boyfriend, and I could not be more proud of how she has turned out.

Poland did not let me down on the adventures and excitement front that I had hoped for when I took the decision to move here. Since I have been here, I have met lots of interesting and different people from all walks of life, including judges, business people, academics, and medical professionals. I have worked in a variety of roles all loosely connected to my English teaching, such as doing video voice overs, organising Polish miners to go and work in Ireland, and of course running my own English language company employing teaching staff of my own. It was here in Poland at the age of 34, that I was finally able to more effectively and consistently manage my illness, meaning that I could cope without either depressive or manic cycles, so disrupting my life to render me incapable of functioning for months (nearly a year on one occasion) at a time. Whether it has been the completely different circumstances and expectations I have placed on myself since living here, or finally achieving the right balance of medication (I now take 1000mg of lithium carbonate and 20 mg of fluoxetine/Prozac each day), or possibly even that I have outgrown the worst effects of my condition, the result has been that I have been able to negotiate problems and pitfalls and accommodate my successes without falling into the cripplingly depressive or overly exuberant states I experienced when I was younger.

After about two and half years in Kielce, I moved to Wroclaw, bought a flat, and formed my own limited company as a means to avoid the complications of visas and work permits, which were required as Poland was not in the European Union at that point (around 2000). Life wasn't all a bed of roses, and amongst all my partying (and there was a lot of partying) I repeated earlier mistakes by indulging to excess over prolonged periods. On a couple of occasions, where illicit substances were involved, I experienced fit like seizures and even blackouts which were pretty clear indicators that I had to start looking after myself better (I was certainly burning the candle at both ends). On one occasion I ended up in a police holding cell, or "drug tank" when I had become overly aggressive at a party (again I would argue as a result of taking cannabis). But I guess what was different was how I dealt and coped with things, despite setbacks such as these. I have never (touch wood) experienced anything again approaching the extreme depressions or manias from before and eventually I did wise up, modify my behaviour and now I live what by any standards would be considered a boring/domesticated life - and it suits me down to the ground.

Yes, growing older, maturing, and slowing up have all played a part in helping me achieve a more restful and calm state of mind (despite the bloody dogs), but perhaps more than anything else, meeting, falling in love, and remarrying has provided the solidity and stable platform I had always needed (and on a previous occasion had found and thrown away) from which my illness can be subdued. M is a phenomenon, she excels in everything and anything she turns her time and attention to, and I am so lucky that has included me. As I mentioned, I rented out my flat in the centre of Wroclaw and we moved into a house that we bought in the suburbs. Our new setting was perfect for starting and bringing up a family, which we have done with our two boys, the oldest was born in 2007 and the youngest followed on two years later. It is with mixed emotions that I can say I have cherished the opportunity to be fully involved in parenting the boys, as of course this is something, to my shame that I failed to do for Jo (although Caroline and her second husband Andy did a far better job than I would have been able to at the time). It wasn't easy and at times it has been a real stress test on my ability to stay strong, but as the years have gone on things have got better and better, and as long as I maintain my medication regime and keep a constant watch on my own wellbeing, I hope things will remain so.

It was a fateful day when I took the decision to sign up to do the TEFL course, when my life seemed as if it had hit rock bottom and the only way open to me was up, or out of the game. It certainly was a turning point and it helped me re-invent myself at a time when the old me was long dead and buried. I am now almost completely retired from teaching, having been fortunate enough to retire from this work just before Covid, as the companies that I was teaching at were closing down. The good years I experienced at Standard Life provided enough of a pension pay out for me to start my own modest investment portfolio and to now be fairly relaxed about my family's financial security, and the much lower cost of living in Poland has been another positive factor in my favour. Moving to Poland, changed my life dramatically for the better. Despite my failed first marriage, for which myself and my illness take full responsibility, Caroline and Jo and in recent years Caroline's second husband Andy, have always been there for me and I think of them as an extended family despite the somewhat bizarre circumstances.

This is not the life I envisioned when I was aged just 18 and about to go off to University in Kent to study mathematics, at the top of my game, seemingly invulnerable and with the world at my feet. Who's life ever turns out to be what they imagined at that age? I could not foresee the trials and tribulations that would befall me only a few short weeks ahead. My illness appeared to come out from nowhere, although given what I subsequently learned about my mother and her own condition, it is likely that it was just waiting for the right circumstances in which to emerge and let its presence be known. Of course, no one person's bipolar illness affects them the same as another person's bipolar illness, and many people will have suffered far greater and with more devastating consequences than I experienced. I have seen figures that estimate between 25-60% of people suffering with bipolar will attempt suicide at some point and as many as 20% will successfully take their own lives. I count myself lucky, blessed, and eternally grateful that I have had people around me when I needed them most, who have shown me such love, care, and patience, far beyond what I merited, to help me get through, survive, and eventually prosper. I continue to live alongside my demon, my partner, my enemy, my friend, my bipolar self; and I trust I will for a many more years yet.

I have written this book as a reminder to myself about how I came to be where I am now. Along this journey into my past I have laughed, smiled, and cried at the story of me and my bipolar buddy, where there is life there is hope (although it may not feel like that at the time).

Postscript

Having read back through this book, I am very aware that I appear to be placing a lot of the responsibility or at least explanation, for my wanton, selfish, and ultimately self-destructive behaviour, on my illness and mismedication. This may be difficult for you to accept, instead inclining towards an understanding of me as a young man with zero self-control, who saw what he wanted and took it, to hell with the consequences and any collateral damage as long as he got what he wanted). I can understand this interpretation; indeed, I suspect many people who know me well, and who I consider good friends, may share this view to some degree. Who knows? I can only tell it as I have come to understand it, with the benefit of distance and hindsight. Before I conclude, I would like to include two further things for you to consider which may give you a bit more empathy towards my tentative understanding of why my life unfolded as it did. The first is my effort at a diagrammatic representation of the timeline of my life to date. This plots the significant/traumatic events in my life, alongside the introduction of medication or critical medication changes, and I believe it suggests at a clear pattern linking my major manic and depressive periods and my mental breakdowns. I appreciate that this is far from conclusive in proving a causal relationship, but it certainly suggests a pattern.

The second thing which I would like to refer you to is an article entitled "The 9 worst symptoms of bipolar disorder we don't talk about"- written by Matt Sloan (a writer and journalist with a particular interest in mental health and wellbeing) in 2018. https://themighty.com/topic/bipolar-disorder/worst-symptoms-bipolar-disorder/ The piece Matt published, presents a series of statements from the personal experiences of members of the bipolar community about those aspects of their illness that are less well known or spoken about. On the subject of hypersexuality respondents reported having random and disturbing thoughts about feeling dirty and unfaithful in their relationships and feeling a compulsive craving for sex which resulted in their unfaithfulness. The article goes on to quote respondents comments on their lack of impulse control and obsessiveness during manic periods, regardless of the self-destructive consequences these brought with them such as uncontrollable debt, loss of partners etc in the pursuit of their obsessions (in my case making money).

In addition to these direct comments from sufferers of bipolar there is considerable academic research available which highlights these lesser known aspects of the illness.

This isn't a defence or a justification, and as I have emphasised, I cannot separate myself from my bipolar me, we are jointly responsible. I do believe though, that despite how much more difficult it is to immediately identify someone who is mentally ill, compared to a more obviously visual physical illness, the behaviours these people attribute directly to their illness are common symptoms of their condition. Intuitively I have come to know and accept this about myself and my illness and I take some comfort from being reminded that there are many others who have experienced and endured their bipolar illness similarly, this helps me to be a bit kinder and forgiving of myself in understanding what makes me tick and my resultant behaviour.

Marcus Maure – July 2022

In this crude chart I have attempted to show patterns in my behaviour i.e. depressions and mania as they relate to significant events in my life and significantly changes to my medication

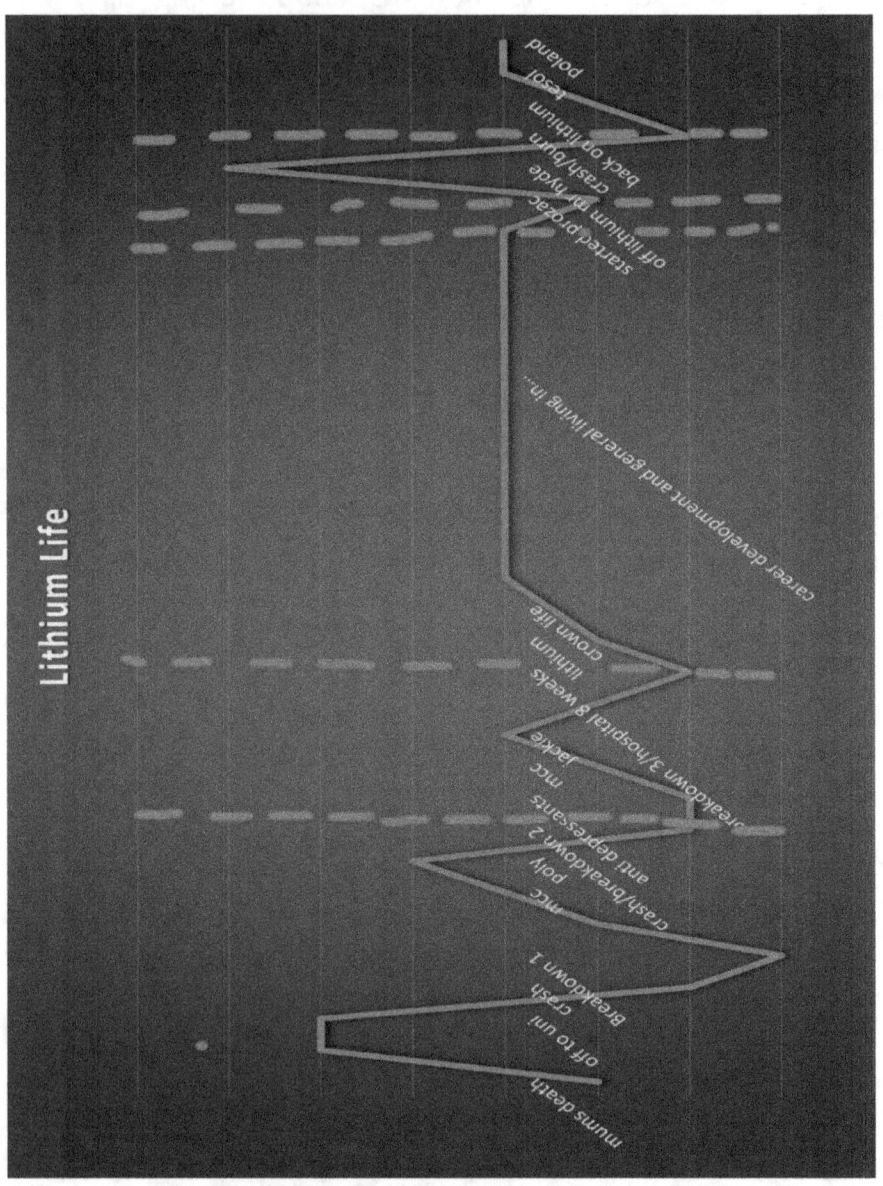

www.ingramcontent.com/pod-product-compliance
Lightning Source LLC
Chambersburg PA
CBHW052349220526
45465CB00003BA/1029